7 DAYS TO A GLUTEN-FREE DIET

. . .

Text Copyright © Deborah Bradshaw, 2015
Photographs Credit: Unsplash.com 2015

. . .

Design & Typeset by Faith Dunbar
Printed by Createspace, USA

. . .

ISBN-13: 978-1519424884

ISBN-10: 1519424884

. . .

Printed in the USA

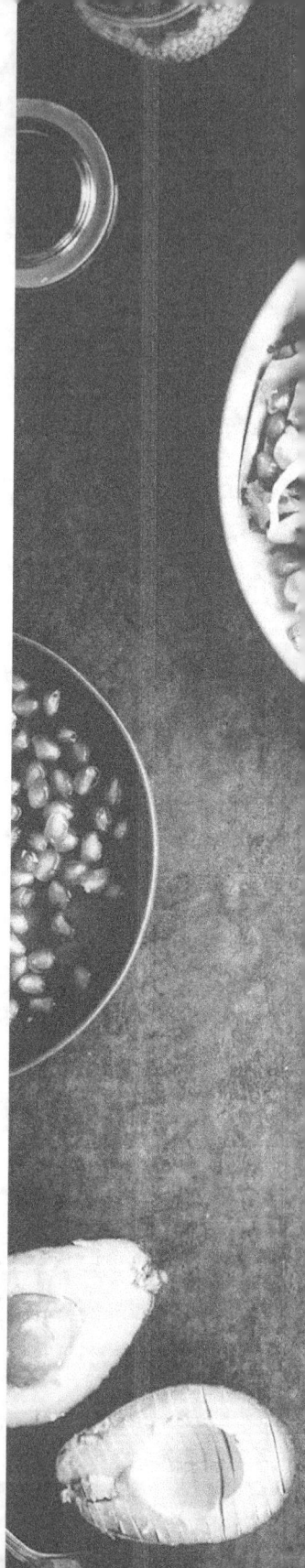

7 DAYS TO A GLUTEN-FREE DIET

A BOOK BY DEBORAH BRADSHAW

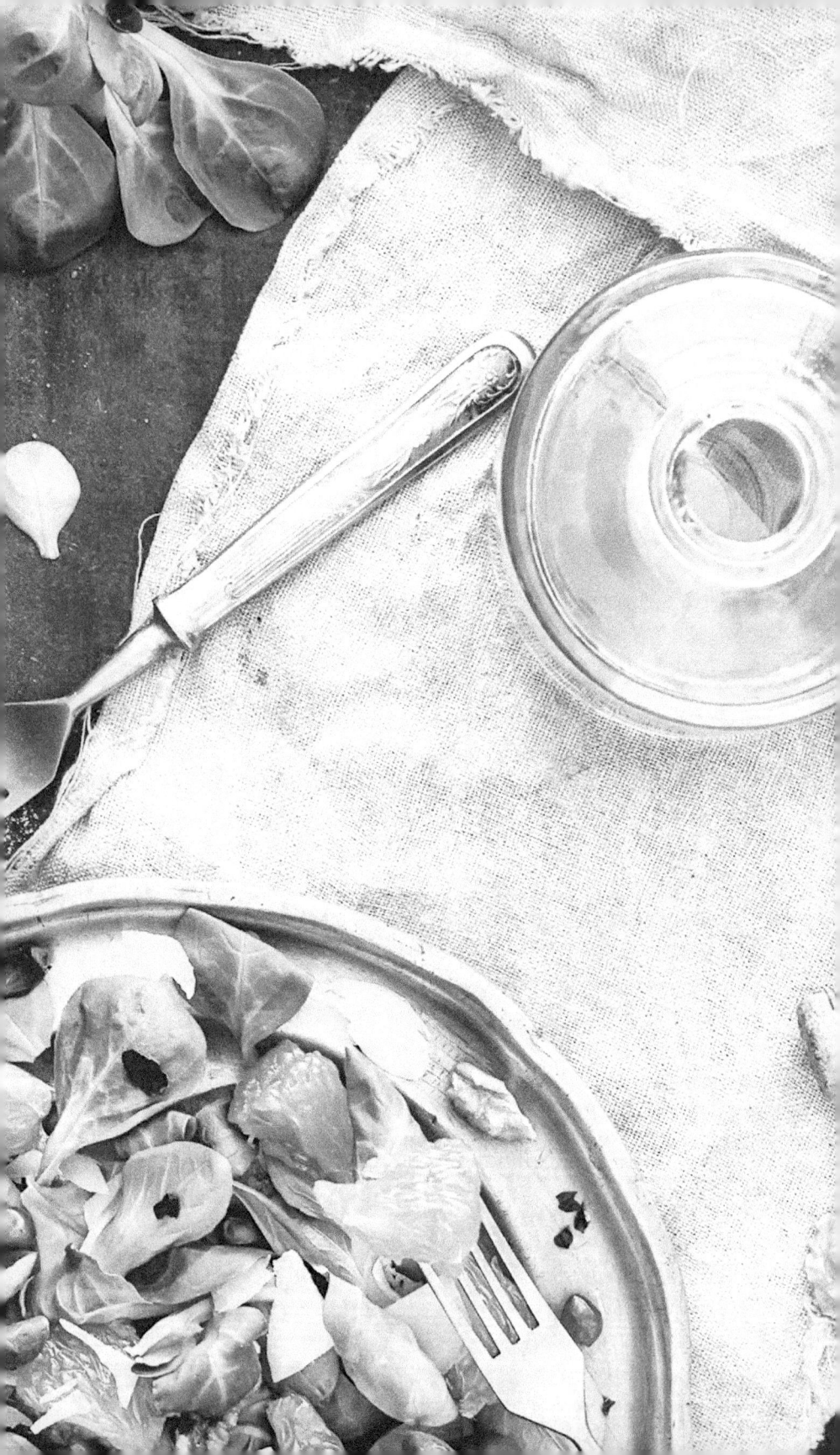

CONTENTS

7 DAYS TO A GLUTEN-FREE DIET

INTRODUCTION

Gluten Free seems to be all the rage. Everywhere you look people are telling you to go gluten free or they are touting a gluten free diet. So why all the interest and why should you consider a gluten free diet?

In this book, we will explore why people decide to make the change to a gluten free diet, how it can be done in a reasonable manner and what steps to take if you want to give it a try. If you want to go "gluten free", this book teaches you how to do it easily and effectively in just 7 days.

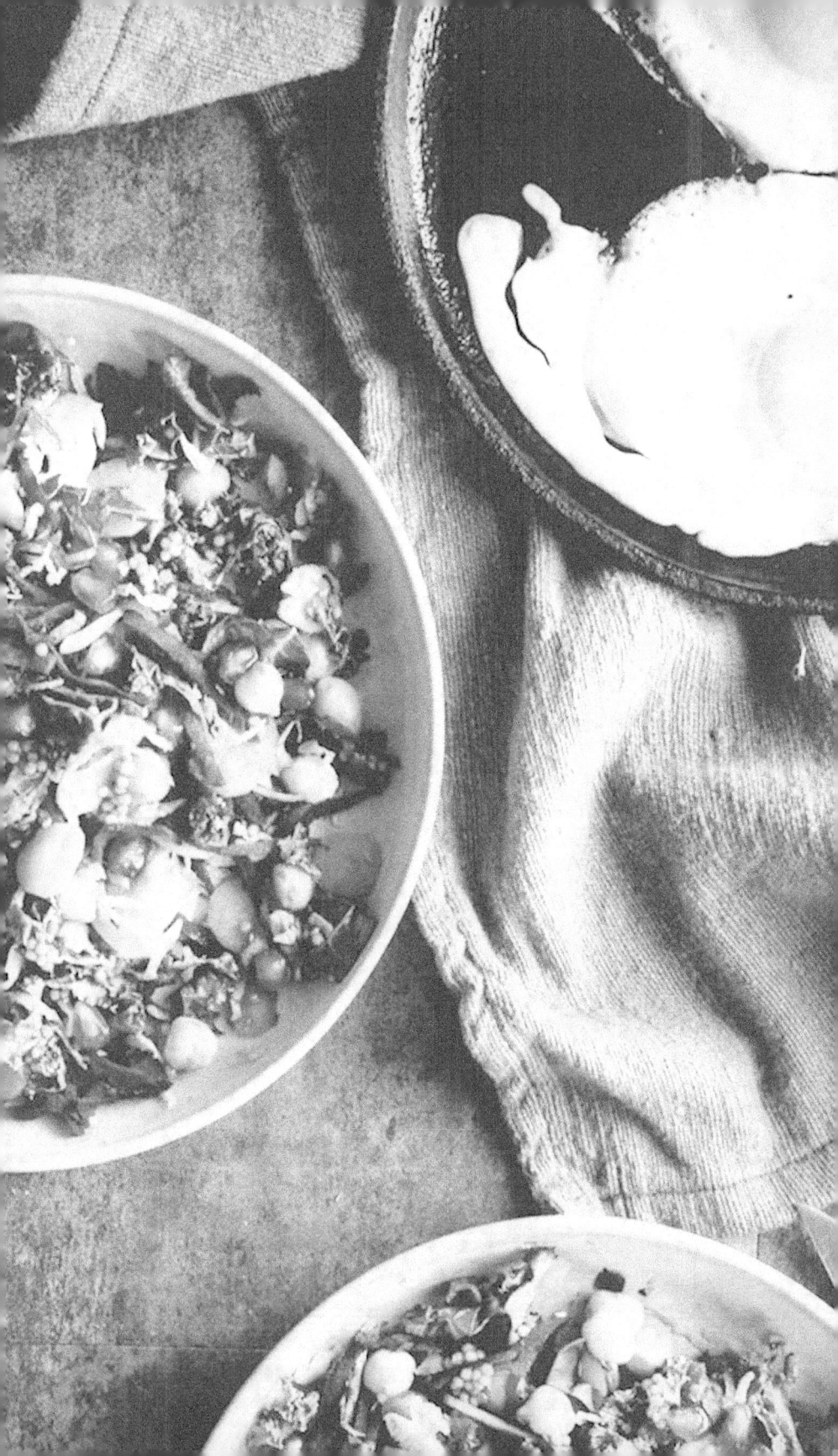

DAY 1

Learning What a Gluten Free Diet Means and Why?

A GLUTEN-FREE DIET IS A DIET THAT EXCLUDES THE PROTEIN GLUTEN. GLUTEN IS FOUND IN GRAINS SUCH AS WHEAT, BARLEY, RYE, AND A CROSS BETWEEN WHEAT AND RYE CALLED TRITICALE.

The usual reason for a gluten-free diet is primarily the treatment of celiac disease. Gluten causes inflammation in the small intestines of people with celiac disease. This inflammation causes many symptoms often mistaken for other illnesses. Eating a gluten-free diet helps people with celiac disease control their signs and symptoms and prevent further complications.

My personal journey towards a gluten free diet began about 7 years ago. I had been diagnosed with an autoimmune disease, but the doctors were still mystified by many of my symptoms. I went to specialty clinics and even went to a psychiatrist to make sure that I wasn't imagining my illness. While they believed my illness was real, they could not determine the cause. In the meantime, I continued to decline. At one point, I was even told to consider getting my affairs in order.

I credit my rheumatologist for being willing to think outside the box, he suggested I consider being checked for celiac disease. The symptoms of celiac disease can be tricky and were just becoming more prominently discussed in medical journals and the symptoms were becoming more recognizable to physicians.

A thin person with chronic diarrhea was initially the symptom many physicians were taught to look for when diagnosing celiac disease. Previously tall and thin, I was gaining weight even as I was increasing my activity level and cutting back on my caloric intake. Also, I had chronic constipation, not diarrhea. My other symptoms included wide-spread pain, muscle weakness, intermittent difficulty thinking clearly, exhaustion, and more.

I wondered if this was to be my lot in life, however all of that changed when I decided to investigate my rheumatologists suggestion of celiac disease. It was through an endoscopy and an intestinal biopsy, that I finally received a confirmed diagnosis of celiac disease. Diagnosis of celiac disease can be difficult but with new information and better education, more physicians are becoming informed.

Although there are many more people that are diagnosed with celiac disease everyday, not everyone who has sensitivity to wheat and gluten will be diagnosed with celiac disease. Many instead have a gluten intolerance. This means that a gluten free diet can still offer benefits and possibly help improve symptoms and lead to a better life. Trying the diet for 4 – 6 weeks, to see if the symptoms improve can be a valid way to determine if the diet will help you.

Some reasons that people are not diagnosed with celiac disease can be numerous and include issues such as the test was performed incorrectly, someone reading the results was not educated properly in the procedure or the elimination of wheat and gluten from your diet before you are tested. You should never eliminate gluten from your diet before you are tested if you plan to pursue testing.

The top symptoms of celiac disease according to the leading websites such as Celiac.com are:
- Abdominal pain
- Anemia
- Arthritis
- Bloating
- Constipation
- Diarrhea
- Dental and bone disorders
- Depression
- Dementia like symptoms
- Fatigue
- Feeling fuzzy headed, unable to think clearly
- General weakness
- Infertility or pregnancy complications
- Irritability

- Joint pain
- Mouth sores
- Migraine headaches
- Muscle cramps
- Nausea
- Numbness in legs
- Osteoporosis and osteopenia
- Pale complexion with no determining factors
- Seizures
- Skin rashes
- Tingling in legs and feet
- Unexplained easy bruising
- Unexplained weight gain or loss
- Vitamin deficiencies

Some experts state that there can be additional symptoms in children such as:

- Attention Deficit Disorder / Attention Deficit Hyperactivity Disorder
- Distended abdomen
- Delayed puberty
- Dental enamel defects
- Failure to thrive
- Learning difficulties and concentration issues
- Severe irritability

There are a number of conditions, syndromes and diseases that some experts believe put people at a higher risk for Celiac Disease. These include but are not limited to:

- Dermatitis herpetiformis

- Down Syndrome
- Juvenile idiopathic arthritis
- Peripheral neuropathy
- Sjogrens Syndrome
- Thyroid disease
- Type 1 diabetes
- Turner Syndrome
- Williams Syndrome

A few of the diseases that can mimic Celiac Disease are:

- Fibromyalgia
- Anemia
- Crohns Disease
- Gastric ulcers
- Irritable Bowl
- Parasitic infections
- Skin disorders
- Nervous conditions and more

In other words, if you have been diagnosed with these diseases, you might consider being tested for Celiac disease. In the article *Diagnosed with Celiac Disease? How lucky are you!,*" Danna Korn, one of the foremost experts in Celiac Disease wrote that "for every person diagnosed with Celiac Disease, 140 go undiagnosed." That means many people who have been told that they will have to live with their particular disease could potentially be helped by a gluten free diet.

So what exactly is gluten? Gluten is a type of protein present in certain grains, such as wheat, that is responsible for the elastic texture of dough. It is actually a mixture of two proteins and in people with sensitivity to gluten, or those who have celiac disease, it causes illness and multiple symptoms.

Some of the most common sources of gluten are: (Please see complete list on resource page #

- Wheat
- Barley
- Rye
- Bulgur
- Faro
- Kamut
- Spelt
- and
- Triticale - a hybrid of wheat and rye

These gluten sources can be in multiple products from the foods we eat, medication or vitamins we take, in shampoo and other personal product we use. The gluten in products other than food is a great source of controversy in the scientific world. Some say that the only gluten that can affect your health is gluten that is ingested. Others say that the gluten found in personal products and shampoo should be avoided as it can be absorbed through skin, a transdermal process. Wheat protein is a common ingredient used in shampoo for its ability to make the hair appear thicker and help retain moisture.

My personal practice is to avoid gluten in all forms due to the fact I seem to be sensitive to the products with gluten and have developed itching and rashes when using products containing gluten. You can determine for yourself whether you seem to be affected by the gluten in personal products. However, anything that is used around the mouth could be ingested and should be gluten free.

Hormel« Turkey Chili With Beans 15 oz ▾	
Nutritional Information	
Serving Size:	247g
Servings per Container:	varies
Amount Per Serving	
Calories:	210
Total Fat:	3g
Saturated Fat:	1g
Cholesterol:	45mg
Sodium:	1250mg
Total Carbs:	28g
Fiber:	6g
Sugars:	6g
Protein:	17g

Ingredients: Ingredients: Turkey Broth, Mechanically Separated Turkey, Beans, Modified Cornstarch, Sugar, Salt, Chili Powder (Chili Peppers, Flavoring), Concentrated Crushed Tomatoes, Oatmeal, Green Chiles (Contains Citric Acid), Onions, Jalapeno Peppers (Contains Vinegar), Flavoring, Spices.

Allergen Info: No Allergens present

Hidden gluten is a problem in many products. While there is an effort to label ingredients in our food, there are still many labels that do not list ingredients in a manner helpful to those with celiac disease. Most companies will state which of their products are gluten free on their website. The are also many apps available to help you determine which of your foods may contain gluten.

The following label is an example of hidden gluten.

This label lists no allergens present but it has hidden gluten. Due to the fact oats are easily cross contaminated in the manner they are grown and can be questionable in a gluten free diet, this product would not be considered safe for someone with celiac disease.

Please see the appendix to find a list of other ingredients that contain gluten. There is also a section that names products that most likely contain gluten unless marked gluten free.

Going gluten free is not about giving up your favorite foods. It is about finding acceptable and tasty alternatives to your previous gluten laden foods. As this issue becomes more well known, more companies are creating tasty products that are gluten free. Recently some cereal manufacturers have decided to removed gluten from some popular cereals. In other words, you do not have to sacrifice your favorite foods to go gluten free. Donuts, cakes, cookies, pasta, etc. are still possible. You can find many acceptable alternatives.

For me, going gluten free has been a life changer A strict but fulfilling, flavorful and varied gluten free diet has given me a new lease on life. I personally have alleviated my migraines, have much more energy, have been able to stop my daily pain medication, and have lost 30 pounds The weight came off easily with the diet and I have been able to keep it off fairly easily. I am clear headed, my nausea and the numbness in my legs is gone and my life is much more enjoyable.

For me, going gluten free has changed my life for the better! I now share my life changing experience with those that have similar symptoms. Often I am asked to assist those who have been told to go gluten free by their physician. My purpose is to help them figure out just what they need to do to have an enjoyable gluten free life. In the next chapters, I will give you a step-by-step guide to help make your journey a successful one. It just takes the desire to want something different and the willingness to begin.

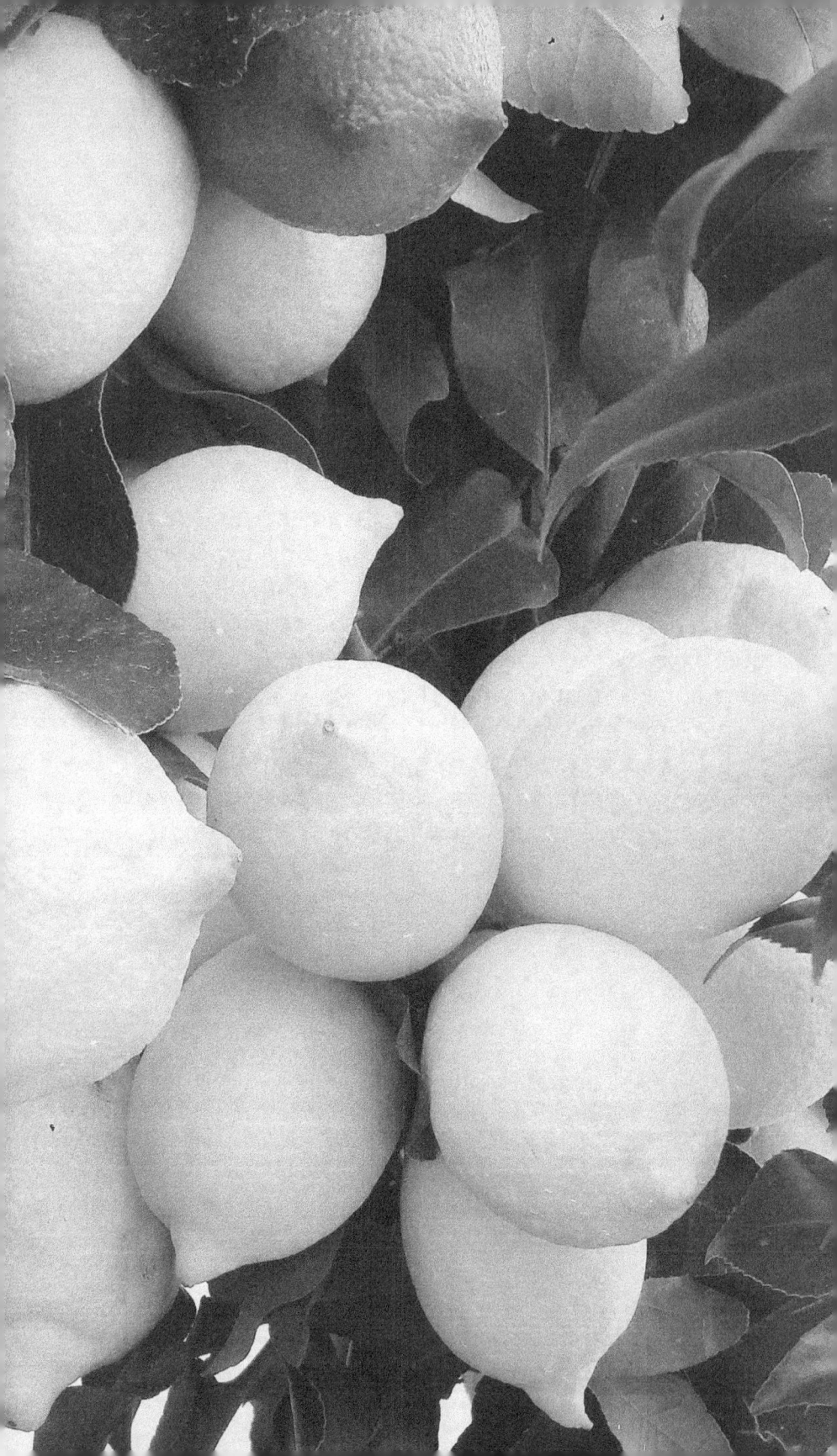

DAY 2

What Does it Take to Go Gluten Free?

OKAY, SO YOU HAVE DECIDED TO GO FOR IT. YOU ARE TIRED OF BEING SICK AND YOU WANT TO FIND A BETTER QUALITY OF OF LIFE. SO WHAT COMES NEXT?

DAY 1: STEP ONE: Who is going on the diet? One of the first steps in going gluten free is to decide if this will be something you venture into as an individual or that you plan to try as a family? If you plan to try it as a family, then I suggest you get rid of the items in the house that contain gluten. If they are open as in a half loaf of bread, you can either give them to a close friend, your local college student or you can just throw them away. Any foods that are not open however, I suggest you either donate them to a local food pantry or to someone who could use them.

DAY 2: STEP TWO: The food. You must determine which foods contain gluten and in which foods you need to consider the ingredients. The most common ingredients that contain gluten are listed in the appendix along with an ingredient list. It still takes some investigation. In the past, it was much more difficult to figure out whether a product contained gluten if it was not obvious. However, today the process is much easier. There are many apps that can help you scan products. Many products are labeled under the label allergens, with any type of gluten they may contain such as wheat or rye. Also now many more products are labeled gluten free, including foods such a luncheon meat, hot dogs, taquitos and more.

Knowing what you can and cannot eat is one of the biggest hurdles to going gluten free. The only treatment for celiac disease, at this time, is a truly gluten free diet. Once you have learned what to eat and what to stay away from, you are much closer to finding success on the road to gluten free.

In the last chapter, the main sources of gluten were mentioned as well as some foods to avoid. Other ingredients that may contain hidden gluten are listed below.

Barbeque Sauce usually states if it contains wheat while others may not. Always double check the label.

According to Breyers Ice Cream, this ice cream is not gluten free but many others are gluten free. They just updated a new list of gluten free ice cream in their brand.

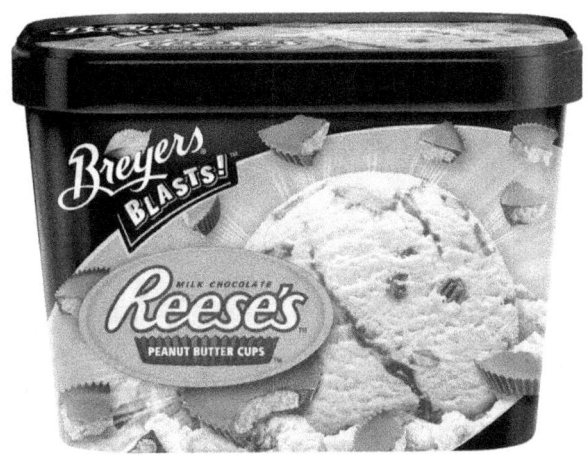

Always double check if something is not labeled gluten free or does not come from a reliable source.

- Imitation crab
- Seasoning packets
- Natural flavorings
- *BBQ sauces
- Salad dressings
- *Hard candies
- *Ice cream
- Chipotles in adobo sauce
- *Yogurt and sour cream (some use wheat or other glutens as thickeners)
- Miso
- Some fermented kimchi

- Fish sauce
- Oyster sauce
- Mole
- *Beverages such as sports drinks or ice tea mixes
- Oats –oats need to certified GF and some people with celiac disease still have sensitivity to oats. Oats in processed foods like chili are not GF and should not be eaten on a GF diet.

Other items that could contain gluten:

- Some multigrain tortilla chips
- Marinades
- Brown rice syrup (It is sometimes made with barley.)
- Meat substitutes like veggie burgers, vegetarian sausage, imitation bacon and any other imitation seafood. They often contain a protein called seitan made from gluten.
- Starch or Dextrin in a meat product, it could contain gluten
- *Pre-seasoned or marinated meats found in the butcher's area of the grocery store or in the meat case
- Cheesecake fillings, some contain wheat flour
- Eggs at some restaurants, which have added, pancake batter to make the eggs fluffier
- *Flavored coffees and teas
- *Some chocolates
- Imitation bacon bits
- Candies such as licorice

STEP THREE: Perception and Understanding

Some of the most difficult obstacles to going gluten free are changing your personal perceptions about gluten free.

1. Getting into a new routine and becoming familiar with the diet.

2. Learning to eat out whether at someone's home or at a restaurant. (This topic will be discussed in detail in Day 6.)

3. Finding which brands you like and personally prefer.

4. Educating your friends and family about going gluten free and why. Again these topics will be discussed more in later chapters.

It is possible to have excellent and tasty food on a gluten free diet. It just takes a little knowledge, a little practice with new ingredients and some experimentation to see what suits your personal and family's taste buds. Make sure to eat a diversified healthy diet. Just as eating lots of processed foods on a regular diet will negatively affect your health, eating lots of processed foods on a gluten free diet will do the same. it is always wise to eat a diet filled with lots of fresh fruits, vegetables, high quality grains and meat.

Grains are definitely still an option on a gluten free diet if you would like to continue incorporating them into your diet. At the end of the book, you will find resources for apps, websites and other resources including my personal favorites of whole grain breads and other gluten free products. Grains that are gluten free include rice, quinoa, buckwheat and amaranth. Even though buckwheat has the word wheat in it, it is not related to wheat, has no gluten and is gluten free. There are other choices but these seem to be the top choices.

Food such as potatoes and corn, while starchy, are naturally gluten free and are perfectly acceptable on a gluten free diet. In order to have a healthy diet, you will want to eat these types of foods in moderation but they are gluten free. This is a good time to not only change your diet to a gluten free diet, but to learn to eat a healthier diet in general. However, the process will be easier on your family and yourself if you include a few of the same type of foods you enjoyed in the past only gluten free versions.

The advantages of a gluten free diet are different with each person. For me personally, the advantages were feeling so much better I enjoyed my life again. I was less tired and much more energetic, including I slept much better at night. In my situation, my body began to heal and several of the diagnoses that I was given were questioned or eliminated. I lost weight and I have reduced the long-term effects of the disease by adhering to a strict gluten free diet.

We still enjoy cake and cookies on occasion and just tonight we had fried squash, a southern dish. Those are the exception not the norm in our diet, however, because we want to stay healthy and watch our weight. Nevertheless, you can now find almost any product you want available in a gluten free version. If it isn't available yet, it probably will be soon. If you live in a small rural area, there are still lots of options. We will discuss those in Day 4 when we learn about shopping.

Many parents who have children with special needs have reported seeing vast improvements in their children's health and behavior when adhering to the diet. Parents have reported such improvements as:

- Better sleep
- Less waking
- Fewer nightmares
- Better speech and speech clarity
- Improved eye contact
- Improved appetites for picky eaters
- Less tantrums and better behavior
- More focus

After being diagnosed with celiac disease, I poured myself into research about the disease. Being an educator by trade, I am prone to research anything I am interested in and my health was definitely something that warranted research. One of the first books I read on the subject was *"Living Gluten Free for Dummies,"* by Danna Korn. I was immediately impressed with her knowledge about celiac disease, her research and her personal journey.

In her book, she tells of her personal journey to find help for her son who was eventually diagnosed with celiac disease. The diagnosis came over 20 years ago when it was much more difficult for people to find out about the disease. Also, information within the medical community was miscommunicated and it was difficult to receive an appropriate diagnosis. There were few food substitutes that were available such as gluten free bread and the ones that were available were in the early stages of development and had an unpleasant taste and texture. I am definitely thankful for the vast improvement in the quality, taste and quantity of available gluten free foods.

In her determination to improve the health of her son, she became an expert in the field and began sharing her knowledge with others. That knowledge was one of the most important factors in helping my son, who has Down Syndrome and was also diagnosed with celiac disease, have improved health and an improved quality of life. As I was reading and researching, I came across a list of the most prevalent symptoms of celiac disease. My son had every symptom. Also, as Danna Korn discussed her personal journey with her son's illness and subsequent diagnosis, she explained her son's symptoms and the hurdles she had overcome to find a solution.

It was if she was telling my son's story, the stomach upset, the constipation, the trips to the emergency room with him as an infant and then as a toddler. At the time of my diagnosis, he was 17 years old, and was experiencing several significant health issues once again.

His moods were changing, he was confused easily, was chronically exhausted, had frequent bouts of constipation and then diarrhea, and had chronic belly pain. Along with other symptoms, he was experiencing significant unexplained weight gain. The closest we came to a diagnosis was when a neurologist declared that he has an unusual case of early onset Alzheimer's disease. It was at this point when I realized he had every single symptom in Danna Korn's book and the light bulb finally went on.

With a diagnosis of celiac disease and a gluten free diet, we saw rapid changes in his health and overall level of functioning. He was suddenly the fun, gregarious, outgoing young man I knew who loved to laugh. His mental acuity quickly became much clearer and he improved in his reading and math skills. His memory no longer seemed to be declining but improving and he lost the weight he had gained plus an additional ten pounds. A short time later, while attending a national conference with leading medical experts and researchers, I heard that some researchers believe that up to 30% of people with Down Syndrome have celiac disease. They also stated that this might be true for other Syndromes as well. For us, the diagnosis of celiac disease was literally a lifesaver.

Going gluten free may or may not have the same effects in your life or with your family but from the many people I speak with everyday who are being diagnosed with celiac disease or gluten intolerance, it is making a world of difference. The biggest challenge they find is in figuring out how to begin. That is why I decided to write this book to explain how you could go gluten free in a logical, step-by-step process. If you do one step per day, then you are only a week away from a major life changing benefit.

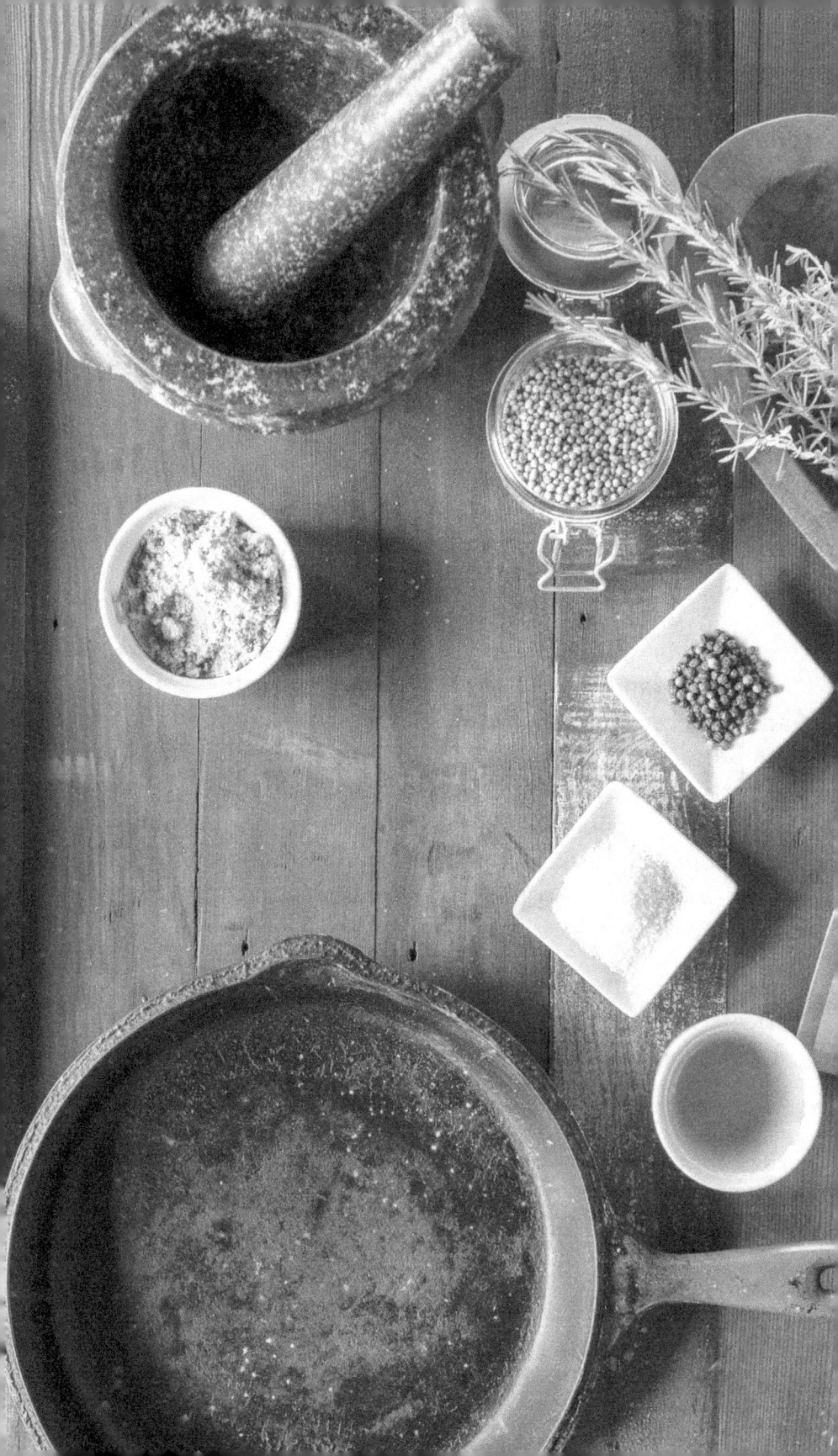

DAY 3

SETTING UP YOUR GLUTEN-FREE KITCHEN

THERE ARE SOME CHANGES THAT NEED TO BE MADE TO ENSURE THAT THE FOOD YOU COOK IS TRULY GLUTEN FREE. THIS CHAPTER WILL DISCUSS WHAT CHANGES YOU SHOULD MAKE IN YOUR KITCHEN.

There are several steps involved in setting up a gluten free kitchen. In creating a safe environment your gluten free kitchen means making sure you limit the risk of cross contamination. You will find suggestions in the following paragraphs but you will also go through the checklist of what you might want to include in setting up your kitchen.

In my home, we have gluten free meals however I have a son who does not have celiac disease and does not choose to go gluten free. For him, I keep a few of his favorite snacks that contain gluten. I also keep a loaf of wheat bread for him. However, he has been educated about celiac disease, the dangers of cross contamination and the need for precautions.

Education of the family member with celiac disease and the other members of the family is vital to ensuring that the diet is kept gluten free.

Do not use any peanut butter, jelly, mayonnaise, etc. that has been used with a knife or spoon. When a sandwich is made, you typically insert the knife into the jar to get the peanut butter or mayonnaise, etc. Then after spreading the substance on your bread, you reach your knife back into the jar to get more. Crumbs are then introduced into the peanut butter or mayonnaise making the product contaminated with gluten crumbs. When you are working so hard to change your diet, you don't want to ruin your efforts through cross contamination. One of the most important precautions we must take in our home are making sure that my son's bread crumbs or the crumbs from anything that contain gluten do not come in contact with our food.

In our house now, we have certain procedures we have developed for using the same jar of peanut butter and mayonnaise. These include squeeze bottles for mustard, mayonnaise and jelly. These are squeeze bottles are available at restaurant supply stores and many times at your local big box or cooking supply store. For peanut butter, we take a clean spoon and spoon the amount we estimate will be used into a bowl. This is them used to spread onto the sandwich. However, in most homes, especially if you are just beginning or you have kids, I suggest totally separate jars of peanut butter, mayonnaise and other ingredients You should also consider keeping these in a different place so that there the chance that someone uses the wrong product is decreased. Also, if you have company or family that comes to visit and is welcome to get snacks and food, then they must also be educated about your kitchen.

Set up separate areas for snacks – those that are gluten free and those that contain gluten. Put them in different containers and store them in a cabinet that has been cleaned especially well to prevent gluten crumbs. Our local dollar store has numerous containers and baskets so when we first went gluten free, I had a color coded system red for gluten free and white for gluten items. I personally used red because it was a mental and visual signal to stop and take notice. White reminds me of the color of regular all-purpose gluten flour and so it was also a clue to the family that those items contained gluten.

In the beginning, while we were becoming accustomed to the diet, I labeled everything. I have a label maker that was fairly inexpensive so everything was marked both basket and shelves to remind everyone where to put the new items and food. We also used the color-coded dots sold for garage sale tags, again white and red. This way there was no confusion, especially for my son with Down Syndrome. I knew he would be reminded by the color if he forgot to read the label. This also works well for children.

Crumbs are the greatest contaminators and one of the greatest issues with having a gluten free kitchen. Washing the dishes well is important but on some types of surfaces, it is still difficult to get rid all traces of gluten. Because of this, I replaced all plastic and wooden utensils that would be used with the gluten free products. While I appreciate high quality kitchen tools, I found my local dollar store to be a great source of reasonable quality utensils and tools. Because any time you are setting up a kitchen and buying new foods and utensils it can be costly, I chose to purchase the initial smaller pieces at my local dollar store.

Colanders, silicone spatulas, measuring cups and spoons, muffin tins, cake pans and wire racks (which I found difficult to clean with no risk of any crumbs) pasta tools, tongs and whisks were all items that I purchased in duplicate to ensure there was no possibility of cross contamination. Other items that should be replaced due to cross contamination are toasters, waffle irons, sandwich presses and the like since it is almost impossible to get all traces of gluten crumbs out of such appliances. Always replace or have a second set of wooden utensils as this is utensil once used for gluten products, it is impossible to make sure they are gluten free due to the porous nature of wood.

If you are going to be toasting any bread containing gluten and gluten free bread, then I strongly recommend a "gluten-free" toaster that you can keep in a separate location. Make sure to educate your family and any house guests as to which is gluten free and which is for gluten products in order to avoid cross contamination. Appliance prices have decreased in recent years and you can often find them for $10 - $20 especially during holiday buying seasons.

When we travel, we often stay at hotels that have breakfast buffets. I usually eat eggs or yogurt depending on the risk of cross contamination. Sometimes however, when selections are limited, I will bring my own gluten free bread.

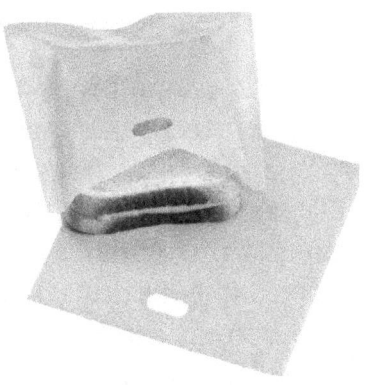

Toaster bags (See above image) have been helpful but you must be careful how you handle them and you must be especially careful with them after they have been in a gluten laden toaster. These are available on websites such as Amazon. While some may consider them controversial, I have personally never gotten sick from cross contamination while using a toaster bag. Mine also came with a set of wooden tongs to help remove a warm bag from the toaster and to keep my hands from the crumbs.

Learning about Gluten Free Baking

Pans with bright shiny surfaces are actually better for gluten free baking because dark pans typically absorb more heat and cook faster than ones that are light. If you only have dark pans, try lining the pan with aluminum foil in order to get even heating and appropriate cooking. Just make sure that you grease the pan especially well if you line it with aluminum foil to avoid sticking. Some gluten free products are more likely to stick to the surface due to difference in texture between gluten free batter and wheat batter.

Temperatures are something that must be monitored more carefully in gluten free baking. Always start with room temperature ingredients, especially liquids, eggs and fats. You need to be aware of your oven temperature which can often vary 25 degrees or more from the setting. This can make a big difference in your final product and so it is wise to invest in an oven thermometer so that you can be sure of the actual temperature. It is also good to know the internal temperatures of baked goods such as bread. Because gluten free batters tend to brown more quickly, it is difficult to tell by the exterior color whether the item is done so the following information will give you a better idea of whether your masterpiece is baked to perfection.

Internal Temperatures of Baked Goods

Yeast Bread – 190° – 200° F or 93° - 99° C

Quick Breads – 200° F or 93° C

Dinner Rolls – 180° - 190° F or 82°-88° C

Cinnamon Rolls – 190°-200° F or 87°- 93° C

Cupcakes and layer cakes – 205°-210° F or 93°-98° C

Molten cakes – 160° F or 71° C

Pound Cake – 210 ° -212° F or 99° - 100° C

Cheesecake – 158° - 160° F or 71° C

Learning to bake with gluten free is really no harder than learning to bake with wheat flour, it is just a different experience. It is an easier learning process to cook with a good premixed gluten free flour and to initially use a recipe that is intended for gluten free baking. One of my personal favorite gluten free flours is *Tom Sawyer Gluten Free Flour*. It is available at www.glutenfreeflour.com. When I was first learning to bake gluten free and especially when I started experimenting with family recipes and favorite recipes, I found the best success with their flour. I now experiment and use different flours depending upon my style of baking but Tom Sawyer Flour is still one of my favorites.

There are quite a few pre mixed flours now on the market and new ones are being released on a daily basis. One of the most important things you need to know about whichever flour you decide to use is whether it already has added xanthan gum or guar gum. Both xanthan gum and guar gum help to replace some of the elasticity that is usually supplied by the gluten in wheat flour. If you do not have one of these gums in your flour mixture, you will want to add it to your baking ingredients, usually at a ratio of about ¼ teaspoon per cup of flour. However, do not add gums to your flour if there is already a gum added. This will make your baked goods have an undesirable texture.

Making sure that the flour you are using in baking has a super fine grind will also ensure your baking success.

You will want to shape gluten free dough with damp hands. Also, a well oiled spatula or spoon can help to shape gluten free dough. Gluten has a unique elasticity that is not present with gluten free goods so learning the "feel" of the bread when it is mixed enough will be part of the learning process. Gluten free dough is more stretchy than elastic and will be thicker than your typical wheat batter. Measuring both your pan carefully and making sure that you have a pan high enough for the bread to rise will ensure your success. Make sure to use the recommended size pan in your gluten free especially when you are first learning how to bake gluten free.

Other baking tips include making sure that you don't try to add too much liquid to your baking especially with muffins. Gluten free flours will not absorb as much liquid as flours made with wheat. Make sure to store your gluten free baked products in an airtight container. I also store mine in the refrigerator. Gluten free goods go stale and spoil more quickly than those made with wheat. Make sure to remove gluten free baked goods from their pan within 5 minutes of removing them from the oven. If you fail to do this, they could collapse as there is more steam trapped in gluten free goods and the residual steam can cause the collapse of baked goods. Always place on a wire rack to cool. Another tip can be adding fruit pectin or gelatin to your baked goods. This can help to retain moisture and give you a product that more closely resembles what you are accustomed to in wheat baked goods. A teaspoon of pectin or of gelatin are usually enough for a loaf of bread but you will want to experiment and do your own research.

Whether you are baking or preparing a gluten free meal, you will want to ensure that your area is clean, free of crumbs and all measuring cups and bowls are also gluten free. Make sure you wipe down the surface and work, area especially well. When I am in a kitchen, such as my mom's kitchen where both wheat flour and gluten free flour are used, I wipe down my work area with one cloth, put it in the washer and wipe down again with another clean cloth. If I know she has recently baked, I may use paper towels initially to avoid spreading any wheat particles and then follow up with the two cloths previously discussed. Do not open anything such as a wheat mix or a mix containing other gluten or any wheat/gluten flours while cooking or baking gluten free. Wheat and gluten flours have very fine particles that can quickly become airborne and cross contaminate your gluten free efforts.

Cleaning and Setting Up the Kitchen

Okay, so let's begin cleaning the kitchen and getting it set up. Allow a few hours for this project as you will want to sort foods, clean, determine what you need to replace and create a shopping list. Get started with the right mindset, you are creating a healthier diet and a healthier life for the person with celiac disease. This is not about deprivation but change, just as with anything there is a learning curve.

Cleaning is one of the most important things you will do to set up your gluten free kitchen. Crumbs tend to hide in drawers, in silverware trays, in the bottoms of containers, on cabinet surfaces, on the stove and in the refrigerator. You will want to wipe down all these areas to start the process of ensuring your kitchen is truly gluten free. You may consider using disposable kitchen and food safe wipes to ensure you are wiping crumbs away instead of spreading them.

When you reorganize your cabinets, if you will have anything that you keep containing gluten, consider putting them in containers with lid to reduce spreading crumbs. Also if you must keep flour that contains gluten, make sure it is stored away from other foods and with a lid so no particulates of flour are airborne. If possible have separate cabinets for gluten free and gluten items. Also if your kitchen is large enough, set up one area where you will deal with gluten foods and another area for gluten free foods. If you must store items in the same cabinet, always put the items containing gluten on the bottom shelf and the gluten free items higher so as not to spread the crumbs containing gluten.

So what do you need to do? Below is a checklist to help you keep track of the steps involved in setting up a gluten free kitchen.

Evaluate

Separate your foods into 3 categories

- Foods that contain gluten
- Foods that are naturally or made to be gluten free
- Foods you are unsure about.

For the foods that you are unsure of you will need to do a little research. Thankfully there are many apps and websites that make this process fairly simple. My favorites are the apps that include a scanning capability so that you just scan the barcode and the app will determine if there is gluten in the manufactured product. Of course, it cannot tell you if there is cross contamination.

Sort

Sort the snacks that contain gluten but that you are keeping into a container, sack or box for the time being. Make a list of everyone's favorite types of snacks so that you will know what type of gluten free snacks to look for.

Determine what kitchen items, pans and utensils that will need to be replaced. Begin your list.

*Please note that any plastic, vinyl or wooden utensils, tools and bowls have the possibility of cross contamination because of the pores in the surface that can trap gluten. Items to replace:

- wooden rolling pins
- wooden spoons, spatulas or other cooking implements
- cutting boards
- strainers and colanders
- plastic utensils, measuring cups and measuring spoons non stick pans, especially those with scratches
- Muffin pans, cake pans and cookie sheets(These can be difficult to remove all traces of crumbs especially if you have had them awhile but it depends on their condition. It is possible to use aluminum temporary pans to bake, they do relatively well for gluten free and can be placed on a heavier pan to produce better results. This can be a temporary cost cutting solution.)

Appliances such as

- Toasters
- Sandwich presses
- Waffle irons
- bread machines

Clean

- Wipe out all drawers and cabinets
- Wash pans and metal utensils that might have had recent contact with gluten or may have been cross-contaminated.
- Wipe down all surfaces including the refrigerator and the oven to remove any possibility of cross contamination.

Make your list

- Determine what types of foods you want to look for.
- Fresh condiments that may have been cross-contaminated
- Favorite snack foods
- Flours and grains that you will cook with – I suggest purchasing a mixed grain gluten free flour that will serve your immediate needs until you learn more about what you like and want to use in cooking and baking.
- Add your new kitchen implements that you will begin to look for.

Educate your family

- Give them a tour and explain where everything must be stored now and why.
- Explain what is gluten free and why it is important to the person who will be gluten free.
- Show your kids the system, whether color-coded or labeled.
- Explain about the toaster and other appliances.
- Explain about condiments and cross contamination.

Demonstrate how to properly clean up crumbs, have them practice and set a new rule that everyone must clean up after themselves.

Consider posting the guidelines for gluten free in a convenient place. If you have small children who don't yet read, this can be done with simple pictures and words.

Tips to a better gluten free process in the kitchen

1. Buy new sponges and brushes to clean with to avoid cross contamination.
2. Wipe down cookbooks that may have flour or crumbs on them if you plan to keep them.
3. Know that for some people with celiac disease a few crumbs can be damaging. **Do not open anything such as wheat flour or a mix containing gluten while cooking gluten free.**

Wheat flour particles are very fine and quickly become airborne contaminating your gluten free efforts

4. Always **prepare gluten free foods first** as to avoid cross contamination.

5. **Don't reuse cooking water or oil** that has been used for any food containing gluten.

6. Wash your hands frequently.

7. Watch out for cross contamination in foods like hummus, dips, butter, cream cheese, etc. Teach your family to avoid cross contamination and start with a new container for the person who is gluten free.

8. Focus–Don't try to multi task especially in the beginning. This will prevent mistakes and cross contamination.

9. Get out a new dishtowel and dishcloth each time to keep the area as clean as possible. Wash dishes and pans well with detergent and hot water.

10. Dry and put away dishes after washing to avoid any cross contamination.

11. Clean out drawers especially silverware trays often to make sure there is no crumb contamination.

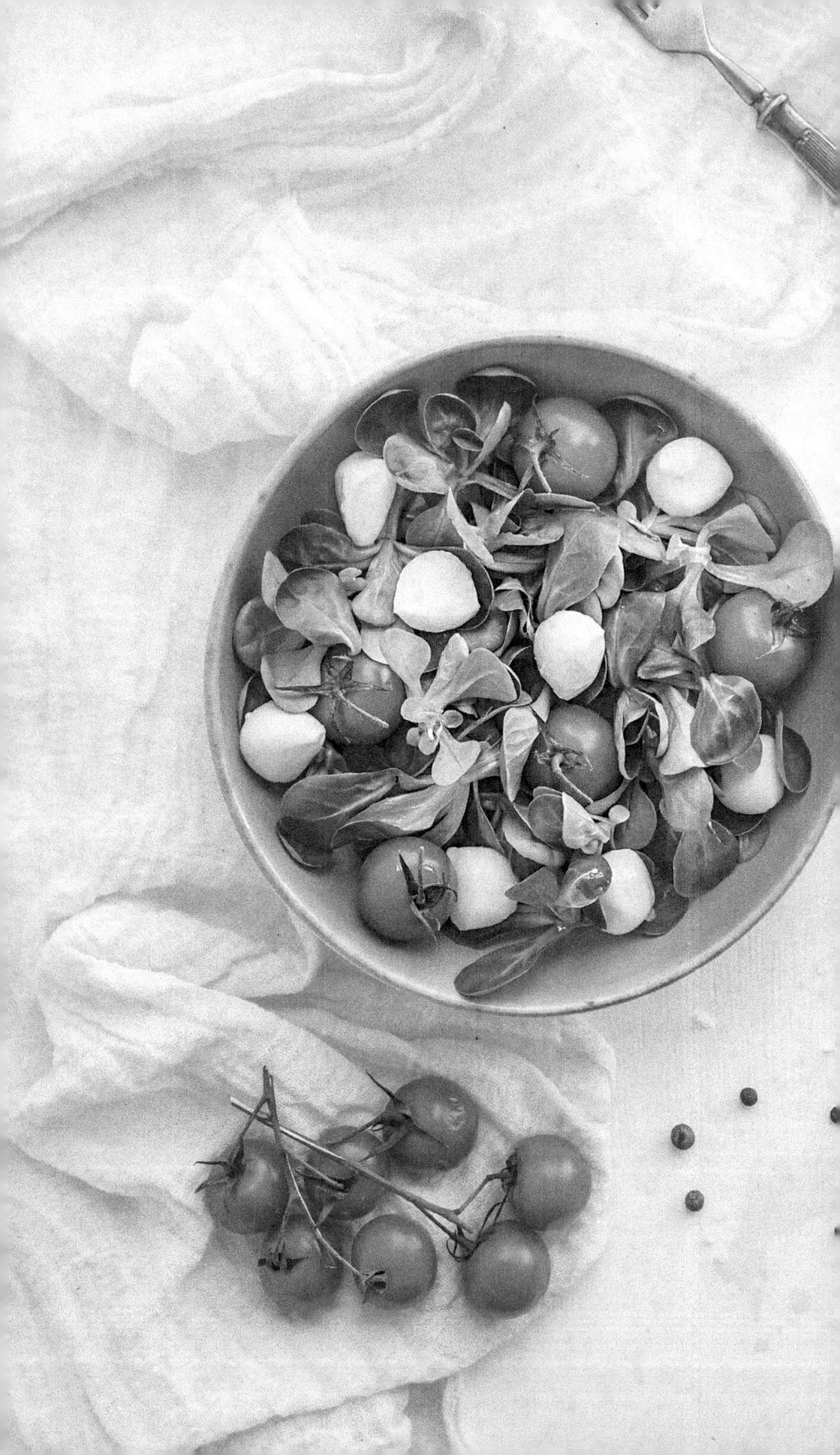

DAY 4

What can I eat?

GOING GLUTEN FREE IS NOW YOUR GOAL AND YOUR PLAN. FOLLOWING THESE 7-DAY STEPS WILL GET YOU THERE BUT YOU ARE STILL A FEW STEPS AWAY.

Keeping a positive attitude and having the determination to more forward are the keys to getting to your goal. You can do this. Just keep following step by step till you get to day 7.

A gluten free diet means changing some of what you are eating not all of what you are eating. So many people think that going gluten free means making a total change in your diet. If all you eat are carbs from gluten and wheat based products, that may be true. However for the majority of people, it is learning what is in your kitchen right now that you can eat and what you should either avoid or get rid of. Here is a list of things that may be in your kitchen right now that you can still eat. Yes, some are junk food but I am listing them because the more I felt deprived, the more difficult the diet appeared.

By knowing I still had the options of some of my favorite junk foods, it helped me get through the transition to a gluten free diet. While my diet now consists mainly of whole foods, it is nice to know there are other foods I can eat if I get a craving.

Junk Foods you can still eat:

(Always check the label as manufacturers are known to change their ingredients but at this time these products contain no gluten)

- Lay's plain potato chips and most other plain potato chips
- Some flavored potato chips – check the label
- Fritos
- Cheetos
- Ruffles (most varieties)
- Tostitos (most varieties)
- Smartfood popcorn
- Doritos Cool Ranch
- Doritos Pizza Supreme
- Doritos Blazin Buffalo and Ranch
- Doritos Taco
- Doritos Toasted Corn

***Doritos Nacho Cheese **ARE NOT GLUTEN FREE**

as are a few other varieties

- Funyuns Onion Flavored Rings
- Jell-O gelatin
- Jell-O pudding

(Many other brands of gelatin and pudding are also gluten free but you need to check the label)

- 3 Musketeers
- Almond Joy
- Babe Ruth
- Bit o Honey
- Butterfingers
- Dove Chocolate (except cinnamon graham and cookies and cream)
- Heath Bars
- Jolly Ranchers
- Laffy Taffy
- Lemonheads
- Lifesavers
- M&M's (just not the crispy ones)
- Mounds
- Now and Laters
- Oh Henry
- Payday
- Raisinets
- Reeses Peanut Butter Cups (always double check the seasonal ones)
- Reeses Pieces
- Rolos (but not the minis)
- Skor
- Skor Toffee Bar
- Snickers
- Tootsie Rolls
- Welches Fruit Snacks
- York Peppermint Pattie

There are definitely others but let's discuss some healthier foods so that going gluten free will make a difference not just in your diet but in your overall health.

Snack foods that we like in our house. I am starting with the snack foods because that is usually what people tell me they miss the most or have a hard time substituting.

- popcorn
- fruit
- Diamond Nut Crackers
- hummus and veggies
- nuts
- applesauce
- apples with peanut butter
- fruit and cheese kabobs
- cheese cubes or cheese sticks
- fruit juice popsicles
- ice cream
- guacamole and chips (most corn tortilla chips are gluten free but again read the label)
- chips and salsa
- nachos made with corn tortilla chips and cheese

*Some pre-grated cheese use products to keep the cheese from sticking together. While most use cornstarch these may also contain wheat, always read the label.

- sweet potato fries (watch the packaging for gluten but there are many gluten free brands on the market)

- edamame
- cottage cheese and fresh fruit
- cheese and gluten free crackers
- kale chips

Of course the number of snacks are probably as limitless as your imagination, but hopefully this list of our snack foods will help you to think about some of the possibilities.

We keep gluten free nutritious snack bars with us when we are running errands and especially when we travel. This solves the issue of needing food when we haven't yet located something gluten free. There are many types of gluten free bars and while your local health food store will have a larger selection, most grocery stores still have at least a few.

Our personal favorites are:
- Lara Bars
- Kind Bars

Foods that are naturally gluten free

- Fresh meats and fish are gluten free unless ingredients are added such as in prepared meats, marinated meats, or processed meats
- Fresh, frozen or canned fruits and vegetables (Again watch for added ingredients that may contain wheat in any processed vegetables or fruit)
- Rice
- Quinoa
- Potatoes – all unless processed

- Eggs
- Milk , Yogurt (most), Cheese (most but watch out for bleu cheese and others that are aged. You can find gluten free bleu cheese) and Butter
- Beans
- Nuts
- Spices especially single ingredient selections (unless they have added wheat or other glutens)

There are others and while this may sound limiting at first, most foods are a combination of these food groups. There are a number of gluten free grains and flours. Again, experimenting a little at time and determining your personal favorites will help you have a rich and varied diet. I have now learned to cook virtually anything we ate before incorporating the gluten free ingredients to make a tasty and pleasing favorite that fits into our diet plan.

There are many things that we ate previously that were actually gluten free or could be made gluten free with only slight adjustments. Below is a list of meals that we make or have eaten. They are gluten free if cooked accordingly. You may have different taste but I hope these ideas will help you start thinking in the correct direction. A few of our favorite easy recipes are also included later in this chapter. It helped me to do some meal planning at the beginning and to have a list of what I was going to eat for the first few weeks.

Here are a few things we ate to help us get started. There are an unlimited amount of cookbooks, magazines, websites and friends where you can get new recipes. Many of the recipes I find, especially those in magazines already are gluten free because they have no ingredients that contain gluten or they can be made gluten free with only minor adjustments. The list is just a few ideas to help get you started.

- Tacos made with corn tortillas, veggies and the meat of your choice
- Enchiladas made with corn tortillas (watch any cream soups, there is a recipe at the end for a cream soup)
- Chicken and veggies stir-fried and served over rice. (Just make sure to use a gluten free sauce)
- Grilled BBQ Ribs, Coleslaw, and baked potatoes
- Grilled chicken or pork chops, mashed potatoes and green beans
- Chili
- Cobb Salad with GF Bleu Cheese or Bleu Cheese Dressing
- Lime Chicken, broccoli and brown rice
- Chicken sausages, pan grilled peppers, and salad
- Pan grilled hamburger steaks with grilled onions, cheddar mashed potatoes and green beans
- GF Pasta, with grilled Italian sausage (cut in medallions) and bottled marinara sauce, served with a green salad
- Rotisserie chicken, baked potatoes and salad (The rotisserie chickens at our local warehouse club are gluten free and so make a quick dinner.)
- Chicken Creole served over rice (Made from the leftover chicken from last night.)

- Homemade Fried Rice (again be sure to use gluten free sauces)
- Pot Roast, red potatoes, carrots and other veggies. (I don't brown the beef with gluten flour and I use cornstarch to thicken to gravy.)
- Red beans and rice
- Frittata with veggies, sausage and cheese, served with salad

There are an unlimited number of meals you can make, some require a little adjustment for gluten free while for other recipes, you will want to make more major adjustments. You can, however, make and eat almost anything you can think about with a little practice. The American diet is filled with bread and sweets. While you can find many substitutions and many premade foods, it may be wiser to stick with a diet that consists of healthier choices of lean meats, vegetables, grains and fruit.

Many ethnic foods are free from gluten. Always do your research.

Here are some recipes that my son and I enjoy. They are easy to prepare and are gluten free. These are meant to give you some suggestions on what you may begin with and to help you think creatively about what other recipes you might already have that either don't contain gluten, or could be easily adapted.

FLOURLESS PEANUT BUTTER COOKIES

- 1 cup peanut butter
- 1 cup sugar
- 1 egg

DIRECTIONS

Preheat oven to 350° F. Beat ingredients together until dough forms. Form into balls and drop on cookie sheet. I actually use parchment paper on the cookie sheet as it seems to help them cook more evenly. Bake about 8 minutes. Let cool about 1 minute and then transfer to a plate or wire rack.

SHEPHERD'S PIE

3 cups homemade or frozen mashed potatoes

In skillet cook
1 ½ lbs ground beef or ground turkey
1 medium sweet pepper, chopped
1 small onion, chopped
2 -3 cloves garlic, minced

When cooked, drain any fat.
Add
10 oz frozen corn or 1 can drained and rinsed
1 8oz can tomato sauce
¾ cup water
salt and pepper to taste

DIRECTIONS

Simmer uncovered for about 5 minutes. Pour into 2 ½ qt baking dish, top with mashed potatoes and sprinkle with cheese. Bake at 350 for 20-30 minutes.

SAUSAGE, BEANS AND GREENS

1 pkg chicken sausage, (I like spicy, andouille or Italian)

1 medium onion, cut into thin wedges

1 can white beans, drained and rinsed, cannellini or northern beans

2 – 3 garlic cloves, minced

1 can reduced sodium chicken broth

About 7 – 8 oz Kale, chopped

2 t dried thyme

2 T balsamic vinegar

1 T oil, preferably olive oil

DIRECTIONS

In a large skillet (preferably 12 inches) heat the oil. Add sausage and onion wedges, cook 6 – 8 minutes until lightly browned. Remove from skillet and set aside. Add beans, garlic and dried thyme. Stir gently to heat and add broth. Bring to a boil, reduce heat and let cook 3-4 minutes or until liquid is reduced till about half.

Add kale a little at a time till all is wilted. Cook and stir 2 to 3 minutes. Add sausage and onions, stir in vinegar. Heat thoroughly and serve.

CROCKPOT VEGGIE SOUP

- 1 – 32oz can diced tomatoes
- 1 medium onion, diced
- 4 – 5 cloves garlic, minced or put through a press
- 2 large carrots, chopped into small cubes
- 2 medium stalks of celery, chopped into bite size pieces
- 2 cups green beans, fresh or frozen
- 6 cups broth (you can use veggie broth if you want this to be a vegetarian dish or you can pair your broth with your meat selection)
- ¼ head cabbage chopped (I have also used Kale but cabbage holds up better.)
- 2 potatoes, peeled and diced
- 1 t thyme
- ½ t oregano
- salt and pepper to taste.1/4 cup balsamic vinegar
- 1/2 teaspoon fresh rosemary, minced
- Salt, to taste
- Ground black pepper, to taste
- 1/4 cup olive oil

DIRECTIONS

I usually sauté the onion, garlic, celery, carrots and spices in 1 T of oil. It adds additional depth to the flavor of the soup but I have also skipped this step if I was in a hurry. Throw everything into the crockpot, cook on low all day or on high about 4 – 5 hours.

I often will add ½ lbs to 1 lb of meat depending on who I am feeding. I like it as a vegetarian dish but I have also added diced ham, frozen chicken thighs or breasts so they don't overcook, or sliced pre cooked sausage links. Make it your own, add or subtract veggies as you like but it is a good easy basic and smells wonderful at the end of a busy day especially in the fall and winter.

Place sprouts in a salad bowl and toss with vinaigrette, to taste. Add bacon or pancetta and cheese and toss again. Season with salt and black pepper, to taste.

Top salad with poached egg and serve immediately.

HOMEMADE TACO SEASONING MIX

- 1 ½ T cumin
- 1 ½ T chili powder
- ½ t garlic powder
- ½ t onion powder
- ½ t dried oregano
- 1 t paprika
- 1 t salt
- ½ t black pepper

DIRECTIONS

Mix together and use instead of taco seasoning in recipe

CREOLE SEASONING

- 2 – 2 ½ T paprika (I prefer smoked paprika)
- 2 T garlic powder
- 1 T onion powder
- 1 T cayenne pepper
- 1 T dried oregano
- 1 T dried thyme

DIRECTIONS

Stir all ingredients together and store in an airtight container.

CHICKEN ENCHILADAS

- 3 cups cooked, shredded or cut up chicken
- ½ cup diced onion
- 4 cups Mexican cheese or Monterey jack cheese
- 2 cans mild green chilies, 1 for sauce, 1 for enchilada filling
- 1 16 oz container light sour cream
- 1 recipe cream of chicken soup
- Corn tortillas
- 1/4 cup olive oil

DIRECTIONS

Mix together chicken, onion, 1 can green chilies, 1 cup cheese. Spoon a few tablespoons of mixture into corn tortillas. Roll and place in baking dish. Mix together sour cream, other can of chilies and soup for sauce. Top enchiladas with sauce. Cover with remaining cheese and bake in 350° oven 20 -25 minutes.

CROCKPOT CHICKEN CREOLE

- 4 skinless, boneless chicken breasts, about 2 – 3 lbs
- 1 sweet pepper chopped
- 2 stalks celery, sliced or chopped
- 1 small onion chopped
- 3-4 cloves minced garlic
- 4 oz sliced mushrooms
- 1 T sugar if desired
- chicken broth, 4 cups of water with 1 tsp of chicken base, or 4 cups of water with 1 bouillon cube)
- 2–4 cups of water
- Salt & pepper to taste

DIRECTIONS

Sautéing the chopped vegetables in a couple tablespoons of oil will help enrich the flavor. I also throw my spices in the pan with the vegetables for a minute or so. This also adds depth of flavor. Add sautéed vegetables and tomatoes in the crockpot. Stir in 1-2 T Creole Seasoning or to taste. Put chicken on top. Cook about 4-5 hours on high or 7 on low. Break or cut up chicken and stir in chicken before serving. Serve over rice.mill). The resulting texture of the leek soup is heavenly – like velvet going down your throat!

Add salt & pepper to taste.

CREAM OF CHICKEN SOUP RECIPE
(FOR RECIPE SUBSTITUTION)

- 1 tablespoon gluten free flour, a finer grind works better
- 3 T of butter
- ½ cup chicken broth
- ½ cup milk (If you are trying a casein free diet as well, you can use almond milk or another substitute for dairy milk)
- salt and pepper to taste

DIRECTIONS

Melt the butter in a small saucepan over low heat. When melted, whisk in the flour and continue whisking until smooth and bubbly. Remove from the heat and slowly whisk in the broth and the milk. Return to the heat and bring to a gentle boil, whisking constantly until the soup thickens. Add salt and pepper to taste.

QUICK AND EASY SWEET AND SOUR CHICKEN

- 1 tablespoon gluten free flour, a finer grind works better
- 3 T of butter
- ½ cup chicken broth
- ½ cup milk (If you are trying a casein free diet as well, you can use almond milk or another substitute for dairy milk)
- salt and pepper to taste

DIRECTIONS

Melt the butter in a small saucepan over low heat. When melted, whisk in the flour and continue whisking until smooth and bubbly. Remove from the heat and slowly whisk in the broth and the milk. Return to the heat and bring to a gentle boil, whisking constantly until the soup thickens. Add salt and pepper to taste.

QUICK AND EASY SWEET AND SOUR CHICKEN

- 3 pounds skinless chicken
- 1 onion sliced into strips (optional)
- 1 20 oz pineapple chunks, drain but reserve juice
- 1 8oz bottle gluten free creamy French Salad

Dressing
- 1 envelope gluten free dried onion soup mix (check packages, some store brands are
- gluten free)
- 1 T grated lemon peel
- 1 small red, yellow or orange pepper, cut into thin strips
- 1 T cornstarch
- 1 T water

DIRECTIONS

Place chicken pieces in a slow cooker. Add onion strips. In a bowl, combine the pineapple juice, salad dressing, soup mix, and lemon peel. Pour over chicken. Cook on high for 3 to 4 hours or on low for about 6 to 7 hours.

30 minutes before serving, add pineapple and pepper strips. Make sure they are heated thoroughly.

Arrange chicken and vegetables on a platter or shallow serving dish. If desired, thicken sauce with the cornstarch and water. Add the cornstarch to cold water and mix well with a fork. Pour into sauce mix and heat. Pour over chicken. Serve over rice.

APPLE CHICKEN SALAD

- **Combine**
- 1 pound cooked cubed or shredded chicken
- ½ cup granny smith apple, chopped
- ½ - ¾ cup gala or fuji apple, chopped
- ¼ cup toasted pecans
- ½ cup finely sliced celery

- **Dressing – Mix together**
- 1/3 cup gluten free mayonnaise (light versions are fine)
- 2 T sour cream (light versions are fine)
- 1 ½ - 2 t stone ground mustard
- ¼ - ½ t salt
- ¼ t black pepper
- 1 T lemon juice
- 1 T sugar (optional)
- If you want to make this a curried salad add 1 – 2 teaspoons of curry powder.

DIRECTIONS

Melt the butter in a small saucepan over low heat. When melted, whisk in the flour and continue whisking until smooth and bubbly. Remove from the heat and slowly whisk in the broth and the milk. Return to the heat and bring to a gentle boil, whisking constantly until the soup thickens. Add salt and pepper to taste.

Mix together, chill and serve.

OVEN FRIED FISH

- 6 fish fillets, mild white fish
- 1 egg, slightly beaten
- 1/c Dijon mustard
- 1 teaspoon dried thyme
- salt and pepper to taste
- ¾ gluten free crackers, crushed (there are many choices of crackers, I find that the ones equivalent to saltines or other round crackers work well. I have also used gluten free panko crumbs which are made from rice and I find at my local Asian grocery store.)
- 2 Tablespoons melted butter

DIRECTIONS

Heat oven to 475° F. In a small bowl mix the egg, mustard, and thyme. Place cracker crumbs on a plate. Salt and pepper fish on both sides. Dip fish into the mustard mixture and then into the cracker crumbs. Coat both sides of the fish.

Place on an ungreased cookie sheet. Drizzle with the melted butter and cook for 10 – 15 minutes, turning fish half way through.

Serve with your choice of sides.

MEAT LOAF

- 1 ¼ pounds extra lean ground
- 1 ¼ cup gluten free oats (Please do not use regular oats. They contain wheat. Some people have a sensitivity to oats even those that are gluten free so you might try some gluten free oatmeal before you make this recipe. You can substitute 3 slices of gluten free bread, cut into small pieces if you are sensitive to GF oats.)
- ¼ cup buttermilk
- 2 eggs, beaten
- 1 ½ teaspoons salt
- 1 t pepper
- 1 t garlic powder
- ½ onion finely chopped
- ¾ - 1 cup gluten free barbeque sauce

DIRECTIONS

Preheat oven to 350° F. Lightly grease a 5 x 9 inch loaf pan. Pour barbeque sauce on the bottom of the pan before adding the meat loaf. Mix all ingredients together well and place in loaf pan. Cook approximately 45 – 50 minutes till done and juices are clear.

Flip over onto a serving platter and slice before serving.

CHICKEN MOLE

- 2 pounds boneless, skinless chicken thighs or breasts cut into pieces
- Salt and pepper to taste
- ¼ cup of oil (I use a light olive oil.)
- 2-3 T chili powder
- 1 T cumin
- 1 ½ - 2 teaspoons cinnamon
- 1 teaspoon cayenne pepper, optional
- 2 oz unsweetened GF chocolate (Most are gluten free but always double check.)
- 3 15 – 16 oz cans of stewed tomatoes, pureed
- 2- 3 gloves minced garlic
- 1 – 2 chopped sweet bell peppers (I prefer red, yellow, or orange. They are sweeter.)

DIRECTIONS

Heat oil in a large dutch oven over medium high heat. Sprinkle chicken with salt and pepper. Cook just till browned, Remove from pan and set aside.

Reduce heat to medium and add 1 or 2 more Tablespoons of oil to the pan as needed. Add your spices and heat until browned and fragrant, about 4 – 6 minutes.

Reduce the heat to low and add your chocolate. Stir constantly with a wooden spoon or rubber spatula. When it is fully melted and incorporated with the spices, add the tomatoes and garlic. Simmer about 5 minutes stirring occasionally and then add the bell peppers. Cook another 5 minutes or so. Add the chicken to the pot and cook just till the chicken is warm. Usually about 3 – 5 minutes. Serve over rice.

CROCKPOT CHICKEN CHILI

- 2 cans black beans, drained and rinsed
- 1 10oz package frozen corn or one can of corn drained and rinsed
- 1 can diced tomatoes with chilies (like Rotel)
- 1 can 16 oz diced tomatoes or crushed tomatoes
- ½ cup water
- 1 packet gluten free taco seasoning (or homemade recipe from below)
- 6 chicken tenderloins or 4 chicken breasts(Since I use tenderloins, I add them to the crockpot frozen so they don't dry out with over cooking)
- Small chopped onion.
- 2–4 cups of water
- Salt & pepper to taste

DIRECTIONS

Stir all ingredients together in crockpot except chicken. After mixing everything together, place chicken on top of other ingredients. Cook on low for 6 – 7 hours and on high for about 4 hours. (The size of the chicken pieces will determine the cooking time.)

Top with sour cream, cilantro, avocado, and grated cheese if desired.

HASH BROWN DINNER HASH

- ¼ - ½ cup vegetable oil
- 1 16 oz package gluten free hash browns (either cubed or shredded potatoes)
- 1 medium onion, chopped fine
- 1 chopped sweet pepper, if desired
- 2 chopped tomatoes, optional
- ½ lb to 1 pound of chopped ham, cooked breakfast sausage crumbled or any other meat you want to add.
- ½ cup grated or shredded cheese.

DIRECTIONS

Make sure your potatoes are relatively dry before you begin. You can thaw them out and then drain them in a colander or you can pat them dry with paper towels.

Heat your oil in a large skillet over medium to medium high heat. Add potatoes and onions, let cook uncovered about 3 – 5 minutes. Stir well, then cover and cook 3 – 5 minutes longer. Add seasonings, meat and chopped sweet pepper. Turn heat down to low or low medium, cover and cook 5 – 7 more minutes. Watch it carefully and check often so as not to burn your potatoes. Remove from heat, stir in tomatoes if adding. Top with ½ cup of grated or shredded cheese if desired.

CORIANDER CHICKEN AND ROASTED POTATOES

- For Marinade – Mix together the following ingredients
- 2 T extra virgin olive oil
- 1 ½ T brown sugar
- 1 T Sriracha sauce (available at most grocery stores)
- 2 t. ground coriander (I buy this in bulk at the local health food store)
- 2 t chili powder
- 4 chicken cutlets or chicken breasts halves pounded thin
- ½ cup orange juice for chicken
- Olive oil
- 5-6 medium red potatoes
- Minced garlic
- Salt and pepper to taste

DIRECTIONS

Pour marinade into a freezer bag and marinate at least 15 minutes per side. Don't forget to turn over the bag.

Heat oven to 450° F. Meanwhile scrub 5-6 medium red potatoes and quarter. Drizzle with 3 T olive oil, minced garlic to taste, salt and pepper. Roast potatoes about 20 minutes, stirring occasionally.

Add about 1 – 2 T of oil to skillet. Heat a very large skillet over medium high heat. When heated add chicken and cook about 5 minutes per side or until done. Remove chicken from the pan, add ½ cup of orange juice, stir to get browned bits and reduce. Spoon over chicken. Serve with roasted potatoes.

SWEET POTATO AND PEANUT SOUP

- 2 ½ - 3 pounds sweet potatoes peeled and chopped
- 1 onion, diced
- 3-4 cloves garlic, chopped
- 1 - piece fresh ginger about 1 ½ - 2 inches, chopped into large pieces, you will discard this later so you want it large enough to find it.
- 1 t cumin
- salt and pepper to taste
- 4 cups stock, vegetable stock for a vegetarian dish or chicken can be substituted
- 1 cup water
- 1 14.5 oz can diced tomatoes
-
- 1/3 cup creamy peanut butter (I sometimes add a few extra Tablespoons)
- 1/3 cup fresh cilantro, plus extra for garnish
- Chopped peanuts, if desired

DIRECTIONS

Combine sweet potatoes, onion, garlic, ginger, stock, tomatoes, cumin, water, salt and pepper to taste in a large crockpot. Cook on high for 3 ½ to 4 hours or on low for 7-8 hours.

After potatoes are tender, discard ginger. Stir in peanut butter and cilantro. Either use an immersion blender (my favorite way) or ladle into a blender pitcher. Process until smooth. Salt and pepper to taste. Top with chopped peanuts and chopped cilantro if desired.

ASIAN SLAW

- **Dressing**
- Mix together. (I usually use an immersion blender for easier mixing)
- ¼ cup honey
- ¼ cup oil, I use canola
- ¼ cup rice vinegar
- 1 1/2 T soy sauce
- 1 ½ teaspoons of sesame oil
- 3 T peanut butter (I use either chunky or smooth, whatever I have on hand)
- ½ t Sriracha (You can substitute another hot sauce if you like)
- 2 – 3 cloves garlic, minced
- 1 T grated fresh ginger
- Salt and pepper to taste

- **Slaw**
- 1 16 oz package coleslaw mix
- 1 – 2 cups shredded carrots
- 1 medium red, yellow or orange sweet bell pepper, chopped
- 4-5 green onions, chopped
- 1 cup shelled edamame, cooked
- ½ cup salted peanuts, chopped
- ½ cup fresh cilantro, chopped

DIRECTIONS

Combine all slaw ingredients. Pour the dressing over the slaw and serve.

TORTILLA CHIP CHICKEN CASSEROLE

- 11oz. GF Tortilla Chips, flavored chips are good as long as they are GF
- 2 Cups shredded, cooked chicken
- 1 can GF cream soup or GF recipe from above
- 1 cup sour cream
- 16oz grated Mexican or other mild cheese
- 1 10 oz can tomatoes with green chilies, like Rotel
- 1 ½ t cumin
- 1 T chili powder
- ½ cup pico de gallo or chunky salsa.

DIRECTIONS

Preheat oven to 350°. Mix together soup, sour cream, half the cheese, the chicken, tomatoes, cumin, and chili powder.

Crush the chips and place half in a greased 9 x 13 baking dish. Layer in the chicken mixture. Add other half of the chips. Sprinkle with the remaining cheese and bake 20 minutes. Remove from oven and serve with salsa or pico de gallo.

MENU SUGGESTIONS

Below is an example of a two week gluten free menu in our house. I added a couple of extra meals in case your family would like different options. Hopefully this will give you an idea of how easy it really is to create a gluten free meal plan. We love salad so often serve one of several types of salad with our meal but you can add whatever sides please your family. It just takes a little experimentation, practice and planning and you will be well on your way to cooking gluten free.

- Chicken with coriander and roasted potatoes*, salad
- Turkey Chili, GF cornbread, and coleslaw (We like Bob's Red Mill GF mix.)
- Sweet Potato and Peanut soup*, fruit
- Tacos with corn tortillas, ground turkey, refried beans, lettuce, tomatoes, cheese, avocado and salsa. (You can, of course, make them according to your own family preferences, that is just our current method.) Fresh fruit in season
- GF penne pasta, bottled marinara sauce, chicken or pork Italian sausage, grilled and sliced and a big green salad
- Pork chops or chicken cutlets with sweet potatoes, and broccoli
- Beans and Rice, fresh fruit or whatever fresh veggie is in season served as a side

- Homemade pizza with GF Venice Bakery Pizza Crusts and a salad
- Kale, beans and sausage*
- Thai chicken curry, rice and fruit
- Crockpot chicken chili*
- Cobb salad (We like to add toasted sunflower seeds for added crunch)
- Meatloaf*, mashed potatoes and green beans
- Asian Slaw*
- Chicken Apple Salad*
- Creamy Chicken Enchiladas*
- All meal suggestions noted with * have recipes included.

GLUTEN FREE PLAY DOUGH ALTERNATIVE

- ½ cup rice flour
- ½ cup cornstarch
- ½ cup salt
- 2 tsp. cream of tartar
- 1 cup water
- 1 tsp. cooking oil
- food coloring if desired

DIRECTIONS

Mix ingredients. Cook and stir over low heat for about 3 minutes or until mixture forms a ball. Cool completely before sealing in a baggie or plastic container. This recipe should only take about 10 minutes to prepare.

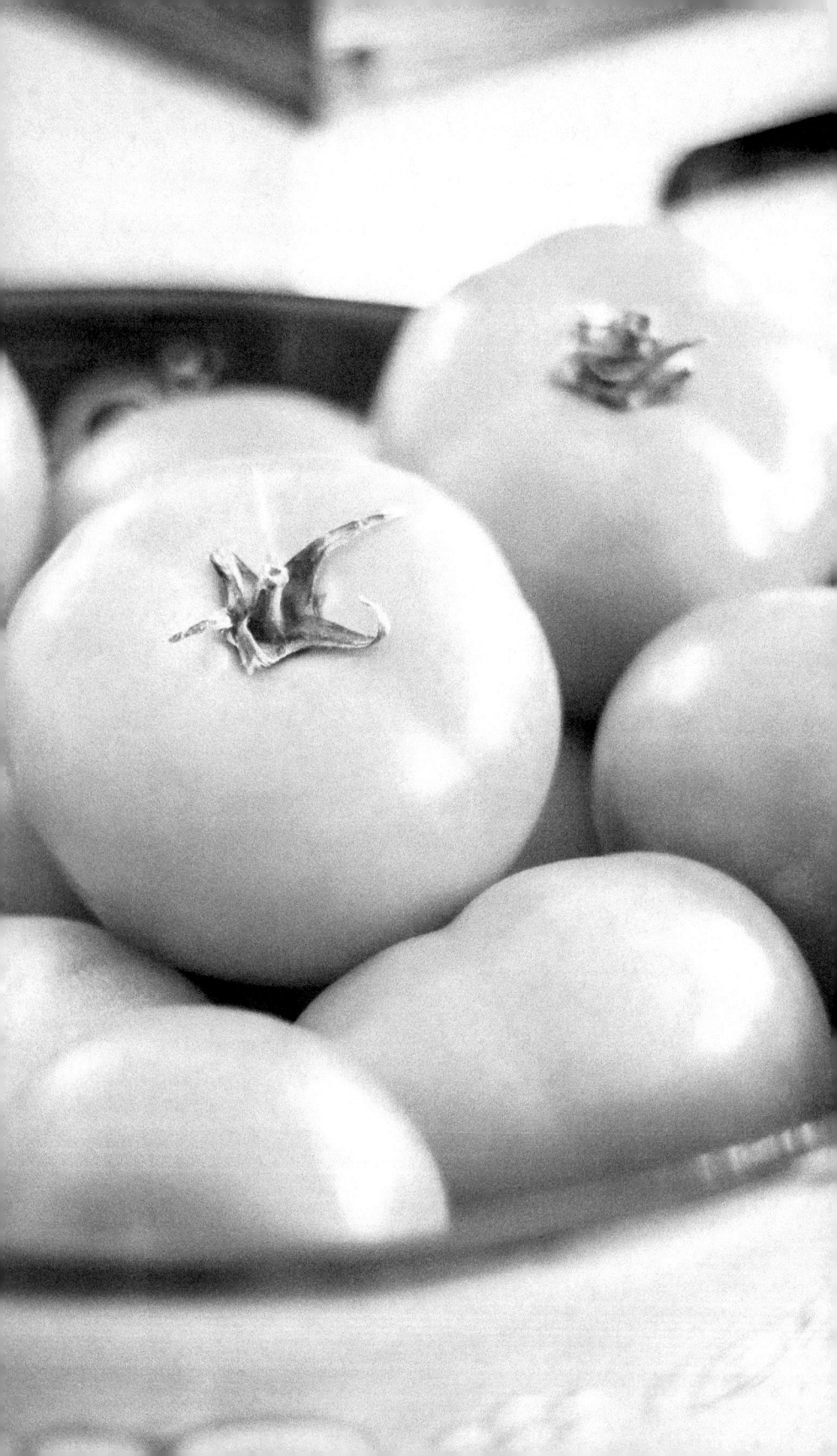

DAY 5

Shopping

HOPEFULLY, BY THIS TIME YOU ARE BEGINNING TO GET AN IDEA OF WHAT YOU CAN EAT. YOU KNOW YOUR OWN PERSONAL FOOD PREFERENCES SO IT'S TIME TO GET READY TO SHOP.

The first thing you need to do is create a list of what you will be buying. Please do not go shopping without a list. There are so many choices it is easy to become overwhelmed.

The next issue is to realize that some items are naturally gluten free. I purchased a $4 jar of mustard because it was the only one labeled "gluten free". Now I know that most mustards are gluten free and the $0.88 jar of mustard would have been just fine. One $4 jar of mustard did not kill my budget however if you are purchasing multiple items and you are paying four times as much per item, as I did, your budget for food can quickly become well above what it needs to be. My own struggle to learn the process is a good part of the reason I decided to write this book.

By following some of the steps that I learned and avoiding the mistakes I made, I hope this will be a much easier process for you.

When I first went gluten free, I was so overwhelmed by the process that I didn't know where to begin. I was not thinking of the process in a logical manner but in an emotional manner. I went to the grocery store without a list and started stocking up on gluten free foods, some that I didn't like, didn't need and many that simply went to waste. Personally, I hate to waste food or money so hopefully this process will help you do a better job than I did with my first shopping trip.

There are so many more selections of gluten free items available than when I began. Gluten free is definitely much more popular than it was a few years ago. Those extra products are both an advantage and a disadvantage. The disadvantages are that we tend to buy more processed foods. We tend to eat more junk food. And it is easier to purchase items you don't really need. The advantages are that if you get a craving for your favorite food, you can likely find a gluten free equivalent. This makes it easier to stick with the diet and makes you less tempted to have just one bite. For many people, that "just one bite" can cause major health issues and can weaken your resolve to stay healthy. For me, gluten is not only a poison to my body but it is addictive. If I have one bite, I want more. By choosing the gluten free option, you are much more likely to stick with your diet.

So what should you buy on your first shopping trip? Below is a suggested list of items you might want to start with to make your journey a little easier. You will want to make sure you purchase another product or replace any item that may be cross-contaminated. You will most likely want to purchase a loaf of bread if bread is part of your regular diet. Also, if you commonly use a lot of flour in your recipes, I would recommend buying an alternative to use while you are adjusting. However, you do not need to do what I did and purchase most of the GF flours available unless you plan to experiment with them all.

So what should you do to make your shopping experience better?

- Create your list ahead of time, know what you want to try and what you need to replace.

- Create your meal list for the next week or so and shop according to the list.

- Set a budget. Give yourself some leeway in that budget but have an idea of what you want to spend. That way you are not shocked by the price at the end.

- Plan to spend several hours shopping while you are getting used to gluten free shopping. Looking and making decisions about new products can be time consuming. Plan to shop at less busy times , if possible.

- Plan to visit more than one store.There are so many options that are available it can be overwhelming, however, I have yet to find all the items I want to purchase in one store. I have a few favorite stores that I shop to get the products we prefer.

- Buy one or two items at a time, especially of new products. Try it out and see whether your family likes it. Then try another. Don't try to buy too many items at once. Pick your favorite and then continue the process of buying a couple of items and comparing until you find your family's favorites.

- Keep a list of brands you like There will be so many new brands that it can be difficult to remember them all, especially if you are sending someone else to the store. A friend of mine actually kept a notebook with page protectors in it. She would cut the label from the package and keep it in the notebook to make shopping with family members easier. If she found a product she liked better, she would either remove the old label, or put it behind the new label in case she had to substitute.

- When you visit any store, whether a big box store or a drug store, make a habit of checking to see what gluten free items they stock. This will give you more options and flexibility with your shopping. Our local dairy and ice cream store actually has one of the best gluten free sections I have seen.

- Once you know what products you like, shopping online can be a good way to find products and save money. Depending on the pricing, sales, and competition in your area, it can be a significant savings to shop online. Plus some of my favorite products are not available in my local area, so shopping online enables me to purchase those products. Shopping online is especially beneficial if you live in a rural area where there is a limited selection of gluten free items.

- Look for gluten free labels on store shelves. Some of the local grocers and retailers in my area mark their shelves with a special sign that says gluten free. This can be a significant time saver.

- Some stores, especially specialty stores, will give a tour, if requested, of gluten free products available in their store. Check to see if your store offers such services.

- Make sure you shop with your smartphone or tablet. If in doubt, you can always look up the item to see if it is gluten free. There are some apps that allow you to simply scan the product barcode and the app will tell you whether the product is gluten free or not. These usually cost under $10 for the app, although there are some free ones. For me, it is worth the money to ensure that my son or myself don't get sick.

- Make sure that you check not only the gluten free section but also the other sections of the store for gluten free products. Sauces and cereals are often not in the specific gluten free section but in the regular section with the other products of similar type.

- Befriend your local grocer and don't be afraid to ask for help. They can direct you to the most popular products and sometimes they will place a special order for you on products you like but the store doesn't carry.

- Don't overlook store brands. With gluten free becoming part of the mainstream, there are often store brands of gluten free products. Several of the big box stores have their own line of gluten free products. At this time, my favorite brand of GF pasta is from Aldis. While you may or may not have an Aldis in your area, I have found we actually prefer some store brands so don't be afraid to try them.

- Give yourself a break. Realize that this is a new process. Don't expect to find the perfect products the first time. Trial and error are the best way to learn what you and your family will appreciate.

- Never shop on an empty stomach, you will buy many more convenience foods and other foods than you are likely to eat.

Tips for making sure your products are gluten free:

- Speak up at the deli counter. Although many meats are gluten free, some items sliced are not. Most stores will have precautions they can take to make sure your deli items stay gluten free. Always talk to the person behind the deli counter about being gluten free. Sometimes it causes extra work for the person, remember to be patient and courteous.
- Shop the perimeter of the store. Meats, poultry and fish are naturally gluten free. Do watch for any added ingredients. Fresh fruits and veggies, dairy products, eggs and cheese are also usually gluten free. (Blue cheese and a few other aged cheeses can sometimes contain gluten because it is sometimes started with wheat mold or bread mold. Look for GF labels on aged or processed cheese.)
- Think about the basics. Beans, frozen fruits and vegetables, and grains such as quinoa and corn are all naturally gluten free.
- Watch for hidden gluten. Ingredients to watch out for include:
- Barley
- Carmel Coloring- If the product is from North America, then the carmel coloring is produced from corn gluten but if it is from another part of the world, it may contain wheat gluten
- HVP or Hydrolyzed Vegetable Protein – watch for hydrolyzed wheat protein in products that

are vegan, vegetarian or have a combination of meat and other protein sources. Soy protein is gluten free.

- Maltodextrin – Watch for the word 'wheat' beside the word maltodextrin.
- Wheat Free is not gluten free - Some products will say wheat free but that does not mean it is gluten free. Always watch for other ingredients that might contain wheat. Unless a product is marked GF, if it says 'wheat free', it usually contains another gluten.

Products to buy for your first gluten free shopping trip

- New condiments that could have been cross contaminated such as:
- Mayonnaise
- Jars of mustard where a knife is used
- Ketchup that may have been cross contaminated.
- Any other condiment like barbeque sauce that either contains gluten or could have been contaminated with gluten.
- Distilled vinegar (except malt vinegar which is NOT gluten free)
- Salad Dressings, if yours contain gluten
- Jelly
- Peanut butter
- GF Soy Sauce if you use soy sauce (Many contain wheat but LaChoy is reported to be gluten free and so is Target's Market Pantry. There are many others as well.)

- A loaf of GF bread. There are many types, it depends on what type of bread you normally eat as to which brand you will prefer. I suggest experimenting and asking friends or looking on blogs and websites about the GF diet.
- An all purpose GF flour for making sauces, etc. I like GF cup for cup flours.
- Cornstarch is a good way to make sauces and gravies.
- GF cereals, bagels or other breakfast items. (My family loves Chex cereal which is almost all gluten free)
- Gluten Free pasta
- A GF versions of a few treats that are on your regular menu.
- Fruits, veggies, meat, poultry, fish and dairy. It is always a good idea to have an idea of what you would like to eat for the first week or so, not just for meals but for snacks.

Check out the chapter *"What can I Eat,"* for some recipes and ideas.

*There are, most likely, many things you already eat that are gluten free. It is just a matter of learning to think about what does and does not contain gluten.

Other Products to Purchase:

- Lip balm, lip gloss or lipstick – anything used in or around the mouth
- A new toothbrush as particles can stick in your old one

- Many toothpastes are gluten free but you need to check your favorite toothpaste to make sure it s indeed gluten free.
- Malted beverages and traditional beer are not gluten free.

Wine and distilled alcohol are gluten free, so are many ciders If these are part of your life, make sure to double check your favorite brands.

When shopping for gluten free, plan to shop places that you may not have shopped at before. Some of my favorite places to shop are the ethnic stores in our area. They have products I cannot find in the other stores that are either naturally gluten free or are certified gluten free. Not every country uses wheat as much as this area of the world. There are many blogs and websites that can give you more information about ethnic cuisine.

Some of the products I buy on a regular basis at my local ethnic stores are lentils from India, rice noodles from many areas of Asia, rice panko crumbs that are certified gluten free, Sriracha sauce, red curry paste, coconut milk and more. One of the things that I purchase is a brand of glutinous rice flour. Ironically, it contains no gluten but the properties that result in it being labeled glutinous work will in baking products. Go with an open mind when you have time to look around and shop at a leisurely pace. Take a notebook to write down anything you want to research or take your tablet or smartphone so you can look it up on the spot. Do your research and see what you find.

Shopping for a gluten free diet does not have to be difficult. Just like anything else you do well in your life, it just takes practice. Go with a plan and hopefully a menu. Expect to have a learning curve on becoming the most efficient gluten free shopper. You can do this, your better health makes the process definitely worthwhile.

Note – When you are in doubt about whether a product is gluten free or if the formula has changed, you can call the company to ask whether the product is truly gluten free. The customer service number is often listed on the product or you can look it up on the internet. There are times when the company will not be able to give you a satisfactory answer, however, I have found most companies to be helpful.

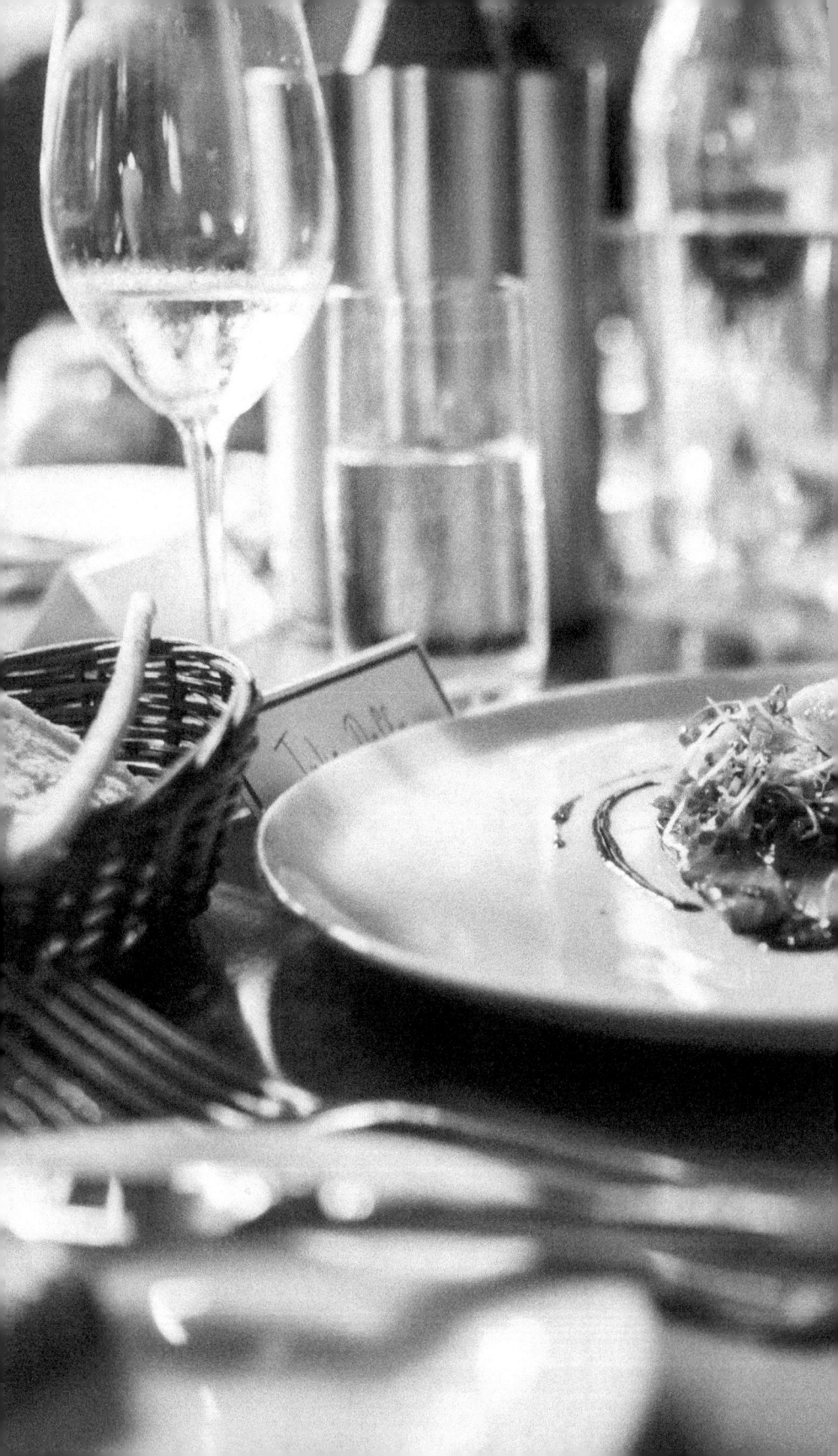

DAY 6

Eating Out

EATING OUT IS ONE OF MY FAVORITE THINGS TO DO. WHEN I FIRST WENT GLUTEN FREE, I THOUGHT I MIGHT NEVER BE ABLE TO EAT OUT AGAIN. I WANT TO ASSURE YOU, HOWEVER, THAT EATING OUT IS INDEED POSSIBLE..

Just like any other skill, it takes a little while to learn the ropes. I cannot guarantee that you will always have a completely gluten free meal. However, with courtesy and vigilance, I can say that my son and I have been sick only a handful of times in the years we have been gluten free.

So what does it take to make sure that your dining experience is a good one? Below are steps that will help you ensure you have the best experience possible. We travel, eat in friend's homes and eat in restaurants. We have been able to find meals that are not only gluten free, but meals that are tasty, healthy and a joy to eat. So how do we achieve this?

Do your homework

No matter where we plan to eat, whether in a restaurant near home or on the road, I always do the research. I find out which restaurants have a gluten free menu or are gluten free friendly. Then I read reviews, if they are available, to see what others experienced when they visited. I look at the menu, again if available, to determine if there are foods that are appealing to our palates. Just because the restaurant serves a certain type of cuisine, doesn't mean your favorite dish will be offered on the gluten free food.

By doing the homework, we have found delightful places not listed on the mainstream websites. Often these places not only understood the gluten free diet, but actually relished serving, good gluten free food. We now keep a list of gluten free favorites for the places we have visited. We look forward to visiting again the next time we are in the area. One word of caution about this, however, is that just because a restaurant has the same name, location and outside appearance does not mean the restaurant is the same. Many restaurants change ownership or management frequently, so always call ahead to make sure that the restaurant still has a gluten free menu.

Can I still eat fast food?

Yes, most fast food restaurants have a gluten free menu or at least a list of items that should be gluten free. One website "Travel the World with Kim" has a listing of menus from fast food restaurants that list their gluten free items.

Where do I find gluten free restaurants?

In searching for new locations and gluten free restaurants, the internet is one of the best tools available. Personally I find that the internet is often better than the apps because there seems to be more information. One app that has been helpful is iCanEat Fast Food but it is only available for Apple devices and can be found in their app store. you will find several other apps listed in the resource section.

Ask around

If you have friends or acquaintances that are also on a gluten free diet, they may be a good resource. Most of my friends enjoy eating out as much as I do and have great tips for restaurants where they have found great gluten free food. Local support groups and health food stores have also proven invaluable in offering good suggestions.

When I travel, I search for local support groups in the area and see if they have an online list of the restaurants that have GF menus. If there is not a specific listing of restaurants, I will often email the contact person for the support group and ask them for recommendations. I explain that I will be visiting the area and would like to know their personal favorites. They usually know where to go as well as where not to go in that area.

Check travel sites

Check travel sites for your local area or for the area you plan to visit. Since the gluten free diet is more widespread and popular than in previous years, there are more restaurants with gluten free options listed on these sites. I have found many of our favorite restaurants in this manner. There are some restaurants that are such a treat, that we look forward to visiting them again when we are in the vicinity.

When calling ahead

Call ahead to get a general idea of what to expect with that particular location. On occasion, when I ask about gluten free, I am referred to a manager or particular staff member that is the most familiar with a gluten free diet and the precautions that must be taken. Ask the name of the person you speak with, especially if they are particularly knowledgeable or helpful. When you arrive at the restaurant, ask to speak with that person. They will be able to guide you through the menu and help you determine the best selections for your dietary needs.

Be specific

Ask whether they have a gluten free menu or gluten free option. In some restaurants, I have been handed an allergen list and asked to order from that. Some restaurants that are truly gluten free friendly will be glad to explain how they make sure their food is safe. Those are my favorites because it usually indicates they know what they are doing in the kitchen. You will find some restaurants that will even display the GF symbol or certification.. Those are usually the best options as most of the time, they know how to prepare meals to avoid cross contamination. If they seem confused about the process, be wary.

Be prepared

Know how to explain your dietary needs in a simple, concise manner. Practice telling a family member or friend about your dietary and be able to give a quick explanation of why you need to adhere to the diet. Don't be afraid to point out that you can become sick from croutons or bread that is placed on a salad and then removed. However, don't be too dramatic about your explanation. In this world of increased liability, some restaurants will be hesitant to serve you anything more than a glass of water if your make too big a deal of the matter.

If you are visiting a restaurant with friends and find there is nothing you can eat, then have something to drink and enjoy the company of your friends. If you are there alone or with someone else who needs a gluten free diet and the restaurant had nothing that you can safely eat, then politely explain the situation, pay for your drinks, perhaps leave a few dollars tip especially if they were trying to be accommodating and leave quietly.

Be patient and polite.

It is easy to become frustrated when you are trying to figure out a new menu and trying to determine what you can eat on the menu. Sometimes you will get a new wait staff who is not familiar with the menu and really has no idea what is gluten free. Occasionally that new person is someone in the kitchen. As tempting as it is to let them know your feelings, take a breath and start fresh.

No one likes to be told what they are doing wrong. One of our most basic human desires is to feel respected and valued. So take a breath, count to five and be pleasant. The person will most likely act towards you the way you act towards them. If you are patient and respectful, they will be also. Ask them for suggestions. If they tell you they do not know an answer, ask politely about whether they could check with someone or you could speak directly with a chef, kitchen manager, or restaurant manager. These people can usually answer your questions and help you to make good decisions as to what will be safe to eat.

Smile and be genuinely friendly.

Ask for help, don't order people around. Remember the time constraint of the wait staff, don't take 10 minutes to ask questions and give instructions. Come prepared ahead of time. Working in a restaurant is not an easy job, a little sincere courtesy will go along way. Don't forget to say thank you and to show your thankfulness in their tip when people go the extra mile for you.

Think ahead.

When you arrive at the restaurant and before you are seated, ask your hostess if you may see the gluten free menu. If you are being seated immediately upon arrival, ask for a gluten free menu. It's better to ask your hostess than to request your server go retrieve a gluten free menu for you.

Ask your server the appropriate questions.

When ordering a salad, ask if the dressing is gluten free and if it is served with croutons or bread. If so, respectfully remind them to please leave those off. Ask about whether the side items might contain gluten. Mashed potatoes may contain flour, broccoli can be topped with breadcrumbs and some vegetables may have a seasoning that contains gluten so always double check. Are the French fries cooked in a dedicated fryer? Is the GF pasta cooked in the same water as the other pasta? Meat, while gluten free by itself, may have been marinated in a solution that contains gluten. You are beginning to understand all of the items that might contain gluten. Always double check, your server may not think to write those accommodations on the ticket.

Always double check your food

Even if you have eaten at a restaurant on multiple occasions and never had an issue, always give your food a quick once over. Recently, my son and I ate at a national chain that touts their accommodations and has a gluten free bun for their hamburger. We have eaten there repeatedly without incident. Their allergen menu is on a tablet, not on a regular menu. We had the tablet, which should signify to the server that there is as allergy issue. Even with a verbal reminder, we received the wrong buns. The server was overwhelmed and the restaurant was understaffed. When she brought us the burger, we were excited to be having a gluten free burger with a bun and we were also ravenous. I did not double check the food as closely as I should have. Also, with the improvement of GF products, many new GF buns look more like the original. We did not discover until a couple of bites in that the bun was wheat. I should have caught it but didn't. The moral of the story is to always double check your food to make sure it is the way you ordered it and contains no obvious gluten. Remember it is your job to vigilant.

Develop a relationship.

If when visiting a particular restaurant, you had a great meal, good service and didn't get sick, plan to become a regular customer. Learn the names of your manager and wait staff. A place you visit regularly, that gets to know you and likes you will be more willing to accommodate your dietary needs. If you develop a good relationship, they are also more likely to offer additional gluten free items and learn more about the gluten free diet. Remember to be gracious for any and all attempts to accommodate you. Kindness is rewarded.

Making sure your kids are safe in their environments

Schools, daycares, and places of worship can be an environment that have many chances for cross contamination with gluten. Many of these environments also provide snacks to children in their care. This does not mean that your child should stop attending these locations, but it does mean some precautions are necessary.

Of course snacks are a big part of the preschool and elementary age experience. While some snacks contain gluten, you will find others are safe. Begin to teach your child what is safe and unsafe. Show them packages and tell them which items will make them sick and which are fine to eat. Visit the grocery store with them and discuss foods, especially in the snack aisle. By educating them on what they can eat, they will have a better idea what to avoid. My son, even when he started the diet, was very quick to learn what he could and could not eat. He knew the consequences of eating gluten and wanted to avoid those consequences at all costs. If he was in doubt, he would rather go without than risk repercussions. Most people, even younger children, feel the same way.

As previously discussed, many items can contain gluten, not just food.

- PlayDoh and most generic versions of this dough (GF Recipe in Recipe Section)
- Paiper mache'
- finger paint
- some paste
- some types of glue
- some crayons, Crayola brand however states that all of it's crayon are GF
- pasta used to string, count or make crafts
- You can find a more extensive list of products that contain gluten on a number of websites.

In the resource section, you will find a letter that you can print or copy and send the teachers and directors of these facilities. There is also a list of safe and unsafe foods that can be given to the facility. Remember that there will be a learning curve. It is up to you to provide suitable substitutes for the snacks, treats, craft items, etc. While this may seem costly or bothersome to some, it is much better than having a sick child on your hands.

Make sure you notify classroom teachers, aides, principals, the supervisor in food service, the after school care program coordinator teachers and daycare providers. These people come into contact with your child, some on a daily basis and need to be notified of what they might expect. They need to be aware not only of the allergy but also what precautions they can take to prevent cross contamination.

Most people want to cooperate, they just need to know how. If you are adamant but also polite and gracious in your conversation, your school or facility will begin to understand and be much more willing to comply. Ask for an appointment or find a time other than pick up and drop off to discuss this issue with them. Pick up and drop off times are usually hectic and often stressful. You need their full attention to make sure they have a complete understanding of the issue.

In regards to cafeteria food in public schools, "Federal law says that the school **must provide allergen-free foods** for a child through the cafeteria service if the parent requests at no additional costs to children whose disability restricts their diet as defined in USDA's nondiscrimination regulations, 7 CFR Part 15b, and that all school staff must follow the child's dietary needs written into the IEP. The school is liable for protecting children and negligence by staff may result in the necessity for a 1:1 aide to keep the child safe in the school environment." This is from the *www.tacanow.org* website. While no one wants to go to these types of lengths, there is a precedent if this type of action becomes necessary for the health and well being of the child.

The TACA website also has a good essential handout for teachers, schools, and parents. It outlines the rights and responsibilities of schools and families in maintaining the GF diet. While the site is directed toward children with autism, the information is valuable and worth checking out for all parents. The link to the handout can be found at *www.tacanow.org/family-resources/an-essential-handout-for-teachers-aides.*

The most difficult part of interacting with facilities, whether daycares, schools or places of worship, is the learning curve. However, with a little time, patience and tact, this can be accomplished. Remember those who work in professions such as teachers, care for your children and want what is best for them. They just need a little help in understanding the process.

Eating in the home of a friend

Eating in the home of a friend can be challenging or easy depending on the attitude and personality of your host and their understanding of the gluten free diet. However, it is not your role to make these people converts to the gluten free way of life. It is, however, necessary to politely inform them of your dietary issues as you don't want your host to spend all day in the kitchen, creating an amazing lasagna dinner for you, the guest of honor, only to find out when you arrive that you are unable to taste even a bite of their masterpiece.

In the resource section you will find a letter that explains your gluten free diet. It will not always be appropriate to give this letter to your host, but in the cases where the host is a good friend or close family member, it may be appropriate to do so. Remember to use your best discretion and good judgment.

You have several choices in eating in the home of a friend. You can graciously accept the invitation with a diet explanation, then take your chances. You can politely suggest that you meet at a restaurant instead, thereby making life simpler for everyone. You can take a foil food packet which will be cooked on the grill or in the oven with everyone else food. You can go for drinks only and explain that you had eaten later in the day. (Unless you know it will be gluten free friendly, have a snack before going.) Or you can stick to relatively safe options, like green salads. Whatever you decide, please be polite. There is no excuse for a rude guest. If you are unhappy with the situation, you can stay only as long as appropriate then politely take your leave.

Most of your friends will want to do their best to accommodate you, they just don't always understand the intricacy of the precautions. Dining in friends homes usually means a fun and relaxed evening. In my group of friends, we have several people with celiac disease or gluten intolerance. That is indeed a blessing. As such, the others in the group are more aware of the issues involved. We put food with gluten and that without gluten in separate areas of the room so that crumbs from the food containing gluten do not cross contaminate. We also have everyone bring something to share. Those of us with gluten free diets, of course bring foods with no gluten so there is always something that everyone can eat. Remember it's not about the food but about the companionship.

Traveling

Before you think, I can never travel again, please know that it is indeed possible and sometimes even easy to travel with a gluten free diet. It is even possible to successfully travel internationally without becoming ill. Because so much more of the world is becoming familiar with a gluten free diet, travel has become much easier for those on a gluten free diet.

The most important thing about travelling with a gluten free diet is to be prepared. Just as you prepare when you eat anywhere other than your own home, you will want to prepare for your travel. Research the city and country where you will be travelling. Make sure to take dining cards in other languages to communicate well with those who do not speak English fluently. Be prepared to be adventurous.

Take packaged food with you.

While there will definitely be food you can eat, finding it when you are starving is not the best idea, so have snacks and bars that are gluten free. You might consider taking some gluten free cereal for breakfast. That way you can be assured of having a good breakfast even if you are visiting a small town. If you are taking cereal, consider taking a bowl and silverware as these can be hard to find if you are in a hotel. If you don't trust the hotels food, you may not want to trust their silverware and dishes.

Research other cuisines

Know which cuisines are predominantly gluten. Even if you are in a country such as Italy, you will find many other world cuisines. Ethiopian cuisine is often gluten free and the flat bread, when prepared in the traditional manner contains Teff flour which is gluten free. Brazil has wonderful breads, made with Manioc flour, that contain no gluten.. Many Latin American countries also have an abundance of foods that can be safe to eat. If you are adventurous enough to be a world travel, be adventurous enough to try foods from around the world.

Always ask questions

Find someone who speaks at least some English or speaks another language you speak with relative accuracy. Ask them how to explain gluten free to a restaurant if they understand the gluten free diet. Even if they don't, you can ask for specific words so that you can at least construct a sentence verifying the absence of gluten in your food. Invariably, when I travel, people will try to communicate with me. Even if we both only know a few words knowing what words to watch for can be invaluable.

Dining Cards

Again, I recommend dining cards. I believe them to be essential in getting the message across. There are multiple brands and options so look around to find what you are most comfortable with. They list, in many languages, the specifics of a gluten free diet which you can share. I have even used dining cards in the United States when eating in a new ethnic restaurant. Dining cards help to insure that the restaurant truly understands what I am telling them.

Blogs are your friend

There are numerous blogs dealing with just about every subject imaginable. Please remember, however, to always double check the information if something seems to be inaccurate. Blogs, just like books, can be written by almost anyone and you can't always believe everything you read in print. If you believe the information may be inaccurate in some way, do your research. See whether there are other reputable sources that give the same information.

Don't be afraid to get out there and live.

Living behind closed doors is no way to enjoy life. Get out there and experiment. You will most likely experience a mishap or two but you will quickly learn how to prevent mishaps in the future and what to watch out for. With research and dedication, you will find that you can eat many different places and enjoy food.

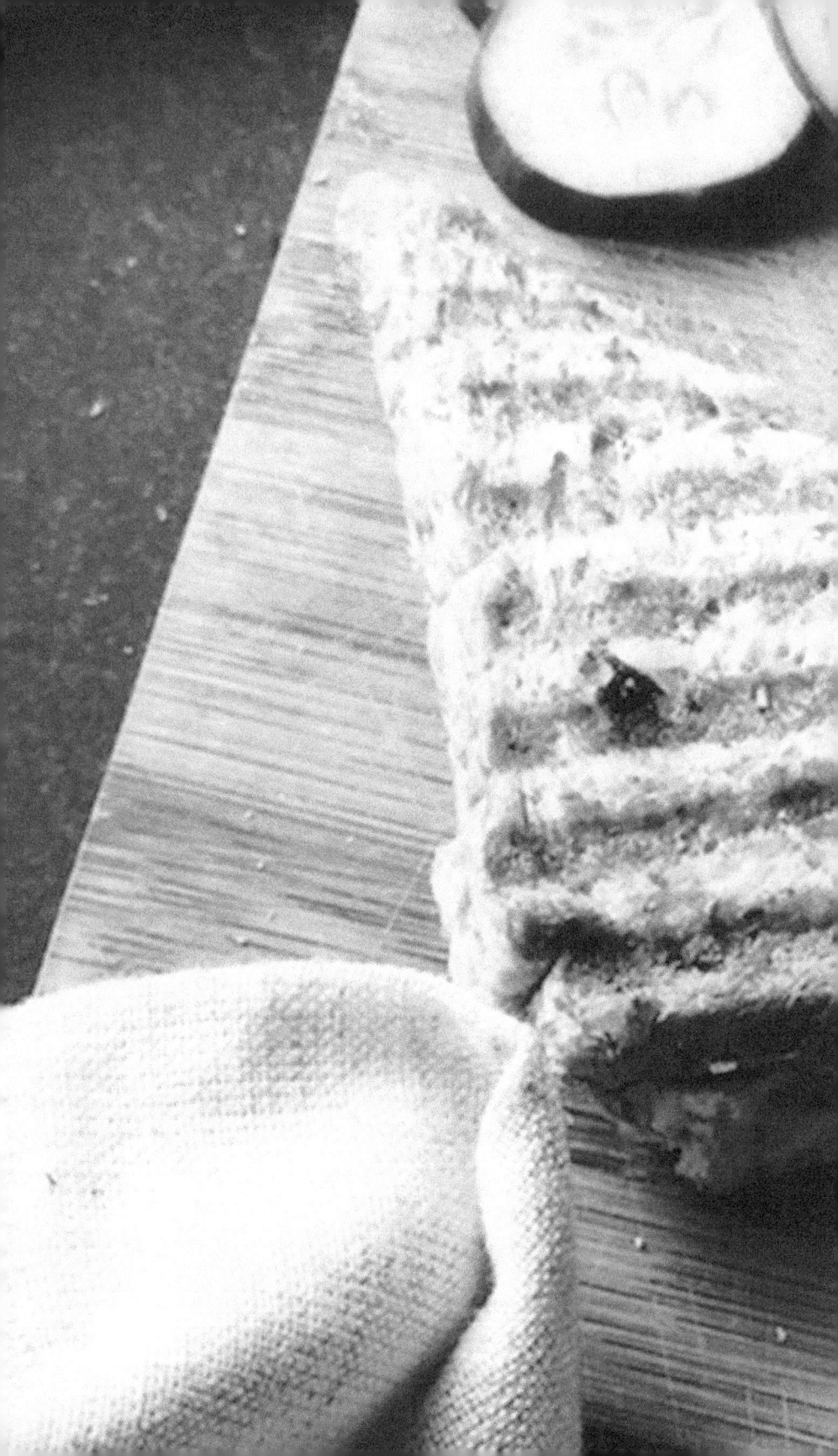

DAY 7

Making the Commitment

My journey was not that difficult in retrospect but it seemed like an insurmountable challenge at the time. However, I knew that I was tired of feeling so sick and tired. I was desperate to have a better quality of life and so I was willing to make whatever changes necessary. My goal in writing this book was for each chapter to lead you one step closer to being gluten free but are you ready?

Where will I find my food?

When it was suggested by my rheumatologist that I try the gluten free diet, all I could think was "I don't know how!" Then, as I waded through the information out there, I began feeling overwhelmed. What would I eat, how would I plan meals my family would like and where would I find what I needed? When I began my journey, there were only a small percentage of gluten free items available in the stores in my area. I did much of my shopping online. However, as the diet has become more popular and as more people have been diagnosed with celiac disease, I can now even find some GF products in the small rural town where my parents live.

I don't know what to eat!

Hopefully this book has assisted you in thinking about what you might eat that is gluten free. I am sure that you will find you already have several favorite foods that are gluten free. Recipes and menu suggestions are included in Chapter 4. These suggestions are not meant to give you a nutritional plan but to give you some options as you wade through the possible choices. One of the most difficult things for me was figuring out what to eat. Many of the magazines that I flip through have a number of gluten free recipes. These recipes are not necessarily labeled gluten free but they have no ingredients that contain gluten. This has been one of my best sources for new ideas of what to prepare.

My family won't like it!

My family knew how sick I had been. They had visited numerous specialists with me and had heard the possible prognosis. They saw me struggle on a daily basis. So yes, they were all for me going gluten free but they certainly didn't want to join me in my new diet. Initially, I tried to cook separate foods for my family and myself but this was complicated, messy and time consuming. We were both dissatisfied and as I was still recovering, this took way too much of my already depleted energy.

As I began to experiment, I initially made foods that needed little or no modification. No matter how you view your cooking or the skill you possess, your family is probably accustomed to your way of cooking. There are most likely several favorite dishes that they have come to anticipate. My family was the same way. I initially stayed away from certain foods because they were too difficult to adjust with my beginner's level of expertise. There were others, however, such as the meatloaf recipe I have given, that continued to be one of their favorites.

By compromising and trying new recipes a little at a time, my family adjusted quite well. Had I tried to move faster on changes to family meals, my family would have rebelled. However, with gradual changes and a continual gentle reminder of why we were experimenting, they did an admirable job, if grudgingly at first, of trying and experimenting with new foods. My family is originally from the south and so I even learned to make a pretty good southern cream gravy and chicken fried steak. By adding in their favorites, my family was willing to take the plunge with me. They still had their snacks and sandwich breads but for the general meals, we ate the same thing.

There is debate as to whether you should go gluten free as an individual or as a family, especially if only one or two members of the family are gluten free. When I was diagnosed with celiac disease, I thought I was the only one in the family but as we soon learned, my son also had celiac disease. Celiac disease can be hereditary and so if one member of the family member is diagnosed with it, it is likely that another member of the family could also have celiac disease. Always remember that if you suspect anyone has celiac disease, they should not be on a gluten free diet before getting tested. The test will not produce accurate results if there is no gluten in the diet of the person being tested.

It's too expensive! Do I feed my whole family a GF diet or just the one person?

So which way is cheaper? You will see arguments for both scenarios, however as I previously hinted, my bias is for serving the same meal to all members of the family. By preparing meals with whole foods instead of processed foods, you will be saving on your food budget anyway. Serving my whole family the same type of meal saved me time by not having to prepare multiple meals. It also saved me money by not purchasing twice the amount of foods I needed for my family. In my house this usually resulted in spoilage of some foods and that was definitely a money waster. No one wants to eat stale cookies.

The cost of some GF ingredients is still slightly higher but we only purchase a limited amount of processed foods not just for the cost but for our health and waistlines as well. As far as desserts and sweets, I usually make them myself as they are healthier. Even though the cost of gluten free flour is more expensive than that of wheat flour, the cost of many GF flours have decreased in recent years making them much more affordable. Cutting down on the amount of breads and desserts we eat, also helps to ensure the diet is healthier and less costly.

Some say cooking from scratch is much more time consuming and I agree if you are cooking complicated meals with several steps. However, I make simple meals during the week and saving the more elaborate meals for when I have more time. By preparing simple meals, I find them to be quick and easy. Having a well organized kitchen where it is easy to find both ingredients, kitchen utensils and pans helps me to be more efficient in the kitchen.

With GF store brands available, I am now able to purchase items such as GF pasta for about the same price as I used to purchase the brand name pasta and my family likes it just as well. When we go to dinner at other people's homes, I always take a dish. Because I disclose that I am gluten free before accepting an invitation, people are aware the dish I will bring is gluten free but I am often asked, "Is this really gluten free?". They cannot believe something that delicious is gluten free. It defies their expectations and impression of the taste of gluten free food. (This subject is discussed in length in Day 6 – Eating Out)

I would also suggest that for my family and me, a gluten free diet has saved significantly on medical bills, travel to those physicians, specialists, and hospitals. The medications, that my physicians have determined I no longer need, have saved me a significant amount of money. Regardless of the money, my health and quality of life have improved enough that it has been worth any cost I may have incurred.

Give yourself a break

Don't think that you have to know everything immediately. It takes time to learn any new skill and learning to manage the diet is definitely a new skill. That does not mean you cannot do it or that it will take a long time. It does mean that you will improve your GF cooking skills as time progresses. It will become easier to read labels and to figure out what your family likes. You will learn new information as you go along. If you feel uncertain or confused, go back through the days and address the issue or seek assistance from someone who is familiar and practiced with the GF diet. For some, contacting a nutritionist can be a good step in ensuring that you know how to guarantee your family is eating the most nutritional foods. Don't be afraid to ask for help.

Be willing to experiment

If you are like most of us, you will have failures when it comes to gluten free cooking. I consider myself to be a decent cook but I have made new GF recipes my dog wouldn't eat. Learning to add the right amount of liquid, learning the little tips for enhancing a GF recipe, and learning whether you need an extra ingredient takes patience and experimentation. It probably took you awhile to become a decent cook when you were first learning. With gluten free cooking, you need to be willing to try something new and to go with your instincts. You will learn what makes a recipe work well and what makes it fail. Be willing to be patient and give yourself permission to take a chance.

Find a support group or person

Anytime you are in a new situation, it is always nice to have someone who has been through it give you suggestions, advice and some empathy. Finding support on the GF journey is just as important as it is with anything else in life. Someone else who knows your journey will help you to be more successful. That person or group can offer you advice not only on the pitfalls and mistakes they made but also on what they learned. They are able to share tips and techniques that helped them succeed.

So how do you find a support group? Today, there are numerous support groups that provide multiple ways to interact. Social media avenues including Facebook, provide access to a variety of support. Many cities and towns have support organizations dedicated to the GF journey. Hospitals and clinics sometimes have support organizations or at least information on the process. Some stores, especially those that carry more health food items, will have classes and seminars that teach you how to cook gluten free. Regardless of where you live, there are options for support, even if it is the lady from exercise class that is also on a gluten free diet.

It is common to find you have friends or acquaintances that are also eating gluten free or that have someone significant in their lives on a gluten free diet. These people will more than likely know of a few good restaurants to get a decent gluten free meal. I have met people while shopping for gluten free items at the grocery store. We often exchange information on good products and good food. Be willing to start a conversation.

Eating together, as a group who are on a gluten free diet, can be advantageous When there are several of you, and you are polite to the staff, the kitchen is usually more likely to remember and accommodate your needs. Not only will your friends have ideas on where to go but they can help you explain gluten free to the staff and empathize with the mishaps that will happen. Just remember to keep your sense of humor.

Check out your sources and information.

While there are many good sources of information out there, it is easy in this day of blogs and social media for basically anyone to write anything and put it on the internet. Remember to check your sources. Do your own research. Just because someone has a long lost relative that is on a gluten free diet, does not mean they are your best source. If something seems implausible, always double check with other sources to see if you find similar information elsewhere.

Consider investing in a magazine subscription or a good cookbook.

Magazine subscriptions offer the latest tips and techniques in gluten free recipes and restaurants. Magazine subscriptions that cater to the gluten free diet list advertisements for new products. This is one place where I actually appreciate the advertisements. It lets me know what new products to look for or request at my local store.

There are a number of cookbooks that are written specifically about the gluten free diet. Some will be to your personal preference more than others. In addition, you will discover some are more informative than others about the gluten free process. If you go to a bookstore, look around. If you are purchasing online, check out the reviews. Ask your friends and acquaintances about their preferences. You will find a list in the reference section of a few of my favorite cookbooks that include gluten free recipes.

This is by no means a comprehensive list but is simply a suggestion of some of the ones my family found useful. There are numerous blogs and other sites that offer gluten free recipes. Again, explore the alternatives. You will most likely find exactly what you need to help you on your journey to eating gluten free.

Look for the GF symbol and learning to read labels.

On some packages the GF label is easy to spot and is clearly marked. On some packages, looking for the GF label can be like searching for Waldo in "Where's Waldo?" Not all packages will have a GF label but all should be marked with the list of ingredients, including those from other countries. You may have to use Google Translate but the ingredients list should be there. As the US and the world becomes more cognizant of allergens in food, labeling laws are changing to make it easier for consumers to recognize allergens and other foods that may not be consistent with their diet. Learning to read the label and being aware of what ingredients to be cautious of is your best way to ensure a product is gluten free.

Keep a notebook whether a digital one or a paper copy.

There are many gluten free foods and brands of foods available. When we were in the experimentation stage, I did not always remember what had been a hit with my family and what hadn't. I remembered the foods we severely disliked but I didn't always remember how the others compared. For instance some baking mixes made decent pancakes but were not our favorite for other purposes like biscuits. Also, because we did not eat these items daily, it was even more difficult to remember our preferences.

A friend who took me on a tour of her kitchen, suggested I keep a notebook of information, tips for baking, recipes learned and favorite brands. This was a lifesaver when I was still learning to shop for our new diet. I kept a list of the foods we liked, however if there were several packages that were similar. I would keep a piece of the package or the whole package that would help me find the product again or to show my friends. On occasion, I would find a particular product at my local store we loved. However, due to the number of new products that are introduced on a daily basis compared with the shelf space at the store, my new favorite product would not always continue to be available. If I had the package, then I could take it to another grocer, or purchase it online. The notebook was also handy for the new recipes that became favorites.

Vary your diet.

As easy as it would be to just rotate the same foods over and over, it is wise to have at least some variety to your diet. Everyone is different and some people would happily eat the same foods week after week. However, to get the maximum nutritional value, varying the foods you eat is a good idea. Vary the grains you use. There are number of gluten free grains on the market that offer various nutritional value. Also varying the types of fruit and vegetables you eat will increase your nutritional intake. While your are experimenting, with creating your best gluten free diet, it's also a great time to add more variety.

Customize your kitchen

The chapter on setting up your gluten free kitchen will help you determine what you need to do to make sure your kitchen is gluten free. However, it doesn't matter how you set up your kitchen if the system doesn't work for you. Make sure you customize your kitchen for the people who will be cooking and snacking in your home.

Find treats

There will be times, especially at the beginning when you are fed up with trying something new. In order to have continued success during these times, have some gluten free treats that you really like. By having a food you love as an option, you will be more successful in the process of adapting to your new diet. This treat does not have to be something newly discovered. In the chapter about what to eat, you will find a list of items like chips, candy and candy bars that are gluten free. This list is meant to help reassure you that you will not lose all your favorites just because you are eating gluten free.

Educate your family and friends

It is important that your friends and family have some idea of what a gluten free diet requires. If you don't take the time to educate them, you will most likely be eating some gluten when your well meaning friends and family make something that is "gluten free." On of the most common sources of gluten contamination is often found in the gluten free food made by well meaning friends and family. Familiarity with cross contamination is essential. Although it may not be the most exciting topic , if they love you and are cooking for you, then talk to them about cross contamination. You could give them the letter to the host which discusses cross contamination. You can find this letter in the appendix.

No cheating!

As tempting as that bite of pie or whatever else can be, please don't cheat. If you have celiac disease, it will damage your gastrointestinal system further. The longer you are on the diet, the more ill you can become from even a small bite. It isn't worth the pain and the health issues that eating gluten will cause.

Stay positive

Your attitude is a big part of the challenge to being gluten free. If you look at it like it's a detriment, if you feel sorry for yourself, if you are always thinking about what you cannot eat, then your chances of failure are high. However, if you look at it as a new adventure, if you concentrate on what you are receiving instead of what you "feel" you are losing, and if you think about the multiple health benefits, then your chances for success are much better. You can do this! Just take it one step at a time and concentrate on the benefits. If I can do it, so can you. Don't wait, reread Day 1 and begin. I wish you the very best with your new life.

RESOURCES

Let me say that there are many resources could be listed l here. There are so many excellent sites and sources that trying to decide what to list was very difficult. This list is purposefully short so as not to overwhelm you. There are other websites that give similar information, these are just the ones that I chose to list. Thanks

GF Support Blogs and Websites

TACA Talk about curing autisim:
http://www.tacanow.org/family-resources/gfcfsf-diet/ - website dedicated to Autism but it has wonderful information about the GF diet especially for kids

Allergy Sensitive Kitchen
http://www.allergysensitivekitchen.com/ -for those dealing with more tan just gluten allergies

Gluten Dude - The Naked Truth About Living Gluten Free

www.glutendude.com/celiac/75-reasons-to-love-celiac-disease - I love his rants

Playing with our Food: gluten-free-girl and the chef

http://glutenfreegirl.com/ - general all around good info on GF

Celiac Chicks - The Guide to a Hip and Healthy Gluten-Free Lifestyle
http://www.celiacchicks.com/ - part travel, part ideas, part food

Art of Gluten-Free Baking

http://www.artofglutenfreebaking.com/ - if you are missing baked goods

Poor and Gluten Free

http://www.poorandglutenfree.blogspot.com/ for those on a budget

Baking Backwards - Food to Live For

http://bakingbackwards.blogspot.ca/ - for the more adventurous eater and great general information

Gluten Free Mom - Just a Mom - Raising her family and sharing what she's learned along the way. Life, Gluten Free

http://www.glutenfreemom.com/ - kid friendly recipes

Travel the World with Kim -Gluten Free and Allergy Free

http://glutenfreepassport.com/allergy-gluten-free-restaurants/fast-food-chains-allergy-charts/

Gluten Free Travel Resources

Gluten Free Traveller

http://glutenfreetraveller.com/ - Reviews of GF restaurants from larger cities and a few smaller ones.

Gluten Free Foods from Around the World

http://www.gluten-free-around-the-world.com/

Gluten Free Travel Is a Thing (And Yes, You Can Still Visit Italy)

http://www.cntraveler.com/stories/2014-12-08/gluten-free-travel-agent-lesley-hock-celiac-disease tips for traveling gluten free

Celiac Travel - Stories and Tips

http://www.celiactravel.com/stories/ - travelling around the world with celiac disease. Specific countries and ideas are listed.

Celiac Travel Dining Cards

http://www.celiactravel.com/cards/ - free dining cards in over 50 languages

Gluten-Free Globetrotter - Your Ultimate Gluten-Free Travel Resource

http://glutenfreeglobetrotter.com/resources/glutenfreetranslations/

Gluten Free Apps to Help You with Determining Whether Products Are Gluten Free

These apps will allow you to scan products to determine if they contain gluten.

Shopwell - Healthy Diet and Grocery Food Scanner App - Free

The Gluten Detective - $1.99

Is That Gluten Free - $3.99

Allergy Free & Gluten Free Diet Tracker - $4.99

Is that Gluten Free - $7.99

Apps to Help You with Restaurants

Many restaurant apps now have gluten free options. Here are some other app options for finding gluten free food in restaurants

Find me Gluten Free - Free

Allergy Eat Mobile - Free

Dine Gluten Free - Free

Gluten Free Registry - $1.99

Gluten Free Restaurant Items - $2.99

Gluten Free & Allergy Free Travel & Trip Planning - $2.99

Some of My Favorite Cookbooks

Some of these are all from whole foods, some use mixes, some are just general cookbooks with easily adaptable recipes. This is only about 1/20 of the cookbooks I love but in the interest of time and money, and because there are so many resources on the internet, these are the only ones I have listed.

- *Cooking for Isaiah* by Silvana Nardone– Gluten Free and Dairy Free Recipes, C
- *The Autism Cookbook* - by Susan K Delane - Gluten Free and Dairy Free Recipes.

- *The Cake Doctor Bakes Gluten Free* – by Anne Byrn - Cakes, Cookies and Desserts from Mixes
- *Saving Dinner* – Leann Ely – Not a GF Cookbook but recipes are easy to make and easy to adjust to make the recipes GF.
- *The Everyday Art of Gluten Free* – Karen Morgan - 125 Savory and Sweet recipes using 6 fail proof flour blends
- *Against the Grain* by Nancy Cain - Extraordinary Gluten-Free Recipes Made from Real, All Natural Ingredients

Letter to your Host

Dear Host/Hostess:

I am on a gluten free diet for health reasons. It is not an elective diet but it is a diet that ensures I stay strong and healthy, not ill.

One of the biggest issues with the gluten free diet is cross contamination. Cross contamination can occur through even minute crumbs. They can be imbedded in a wooden cutting board, leftover from when someone at a sandwich too close to the clean dishes, from a cake that left behind a crumb in the pan or in a jar such as peanut butter or mayonnaise where someone making a sandwich, put the knife back in the jar to get more after spreading the first portion on the sandwich.

There is also hidden gluten in many ingredients including salad dressings, canned chili, prepared foods, vinegar and so much more. Wheat free does not mean gluten free. Please understand that for me, even a small bite of something containing gluten can make me ill for days.

Thank you for your kind invitation. I truly appreciate your efforts and your hospitality. I appreciate being welcomed into your home. Please don't be offended if I choose not to eat or feel I cannot safely eat. It is a process to learn the precautions of a gluten free diet.

For that reason, I would appreciate being excused from eating. Perhaps you would not mind if I brought my food with me. If you would kindly share the menu with me, I will do my best to bring something similar.

I am coming to enjoy your company. While I appreciate the food, you are the reason I would like to attend. Thank you so much for your kind invitation and for your understanding of my situation. If this would make you uncomfortable, I would gladly meet you out for dinner or in my home at a later date.

Thank you for your hospitality and for taking the time to understand my situation. I look forward to seeing you soon.

Sincerely

Things you should tell your family

- This diet is really not a choice. I am eating this way to stop being sick and to start being healthy.
- Please be supportive. I really need your support.
- My whole life may be changed with my diet and precautions but I am doing the best I can.
- Wheat free does not mean gluten free.
- I appreciate the food you have prepared. I appreciate the work you went to in order to prepare me this meal. Please understand I would happily eat it if I could.
- Many items contain hidden gluten, please know that even though they may appear not to contain wheat, I still may be unable to eat some foods.
- Cross contamination is one of my biggest battles. I cannot use the mayonnaise, mustard, (if in a jar) peanut butter, jelly and other things that have been opened and used in the kitchen. The risk of my getting sick is just too great.
- Dishes that are washed with a kitchen sponge can cause gluten to be left or placed on the dishes. Because sponges are porous, they can trap particles of gluten.
- If you visit family and these are not people with who you share a home - I'd be happy to help you learn more about gluten free safety in the kitchen if you are interested, however I know

that the changes can seem challenging so it is your choice. I will not hold it against you if you feel it is too much for you.

- If you live in the home with other family – I appreciate you taking the time to learn the new precautions we must take to keep the kitchen gluten free. I don't want to be ill because I enjoy spending time with you. Illness takes away from that time.
- If I am really craving a certain type of food, please be considerate in your eating of that food.
- Thank you for loving me enough to read this and to learn what you can about the gluten free diet.

Letter to your Child's School, Teacher and Cafeteria Service

My child_____has recently been diagnosed with celiac disease or gluten intolerance. This will mean some changes in his/her diet and in the environment. We sincerely appreciate your cooperation in making sure _____ stays well.

Listed are some precautions and information you need to know. Thank you for taking the time to read, understand and implement these changes. I realize it will be a learning curve for all of us but your cooperation and understanding is greatly appreciated.

Eating

Please have _____wash their hands or use wet wipes before eating.

Please wash the table or have an adult wipe the table before my child eats at the table. Contamination from crumbs either from craft supplies or from food can make them ill.

If you are opening a package for my child of gluten free food, please wash your hands before doing so, otherwise cross contamination could make them sick.

Please, NEVER give my child food or a snack of any type without first verifying it is gluten free.

I would be glad to send party foods or special snacks for birthdays and other special occasions. Please let me know when these will occur and I will be responsible for sending snacks.

I have included a list of safe, gluten free snacks that you may serve. This list will help you verify that the food is gluten free and safe before serving it.

Symptoms

Intolerance to gluten does not present itself like a peanut or other allergy. Anaphylaxis does not usually occur. Below is a list of possible symptoms.

If my child ingests gluten, there are several symptoms you need to watch for.

Please let me know if these occur.

- Bloating, cramps, and foul smelling gas
- Diarrhea
- Constipation
- Severe or medium abdominal pain
- Vomiting
- Irritability or short term memory issues
- Any unusual symptoms or behaviors

Crafts

Many crafts and other classroom products may contain gluten. Some items that contain gluten are:

- Playdoh (A safe alternative is Crayola Model magic clay , however, Crayola Dough contains gluten)
- Papier Mache
- FingerPaint
- Pasta used in crafts and art projects (Unless specified gluten free.)

Items that may contain gluten are:

- Crayons
- Glue especially paste
- Any pasta used in crafts
- Some candy and gum
- Stamps that are licked
- Envelopes that are licked and made outside the USA and Canada
- Ink pads

Please let me know what you will be using and we will work together to come up with safe alternatives.

Obvious foods with gluten include:
Breads, pastries, doughnuts, many cereals, cupcakes, cookies, pretzels, graham crackers, pancakes, waffles, pasta, spaghetti, buns, poptarts, pie, gravy.

SAFE CHOICES FOR GF SNACKS

Many snacks now have a GF for gluten free or will list gluten free on the back. If something is not on this list, you can always double check the package. This list is meant to give you some ideas of what is safe.

Snacks

- Doritos Cool Ranch
- Cheetos
- Mission Tortilla Chips
- Lays plain potato chips
- Act II Popcorn
- Jiffy Pop Popcorn
- Crunch and Munch
- Jello brand gelatin and pudding
- Del Monte pudding cups
- Kraft, Frigo/ Sargento Cheese Sticks
- Nabisco and Welches Fruit Snacks
- Sunkist Fruit Rolls

Candy

- Farley's gummy bears
- Favorite gummy bears
- Trolli gummy bears
- Lifesaver gummies
- Hershey kisses
- Hershey milk chocolate (Not cookies and cream or crispie)
- M&M's (except crispy)
- Nestle's Butterfingers
- Raisinets
- Reese's Peanut Butter Cups
- 3 Musketter's
- Baby Ruth
- Snickers
- Clark Bars
- Dove

Other Candies

- Tootsie Rolls
- Tootsie Pops
- Jolly Ranchers
- Topps Ring Pops
- Pez
- Smarties
- Sweet Tarts
- Starburst
- All Wrigley gum
- Double Bubble

- All Trident Gum
- Dentyne

There are many others. This is just a partial list to give you some ideas.

The following ingredients contain gluten:

- Atta
- Barley
- Beer
- Brewer's yeast
- Bulgur
- Couscous
- Durum
- Einkorn
- Emmer
- Faro
- Farina
- Filler
- Fu
- Graham flour
- Kamut
- Malt
- Malt extract
- Malt flavoring
- Malt syrup
- Malt vinegar
- Matzo
- Matzo meal
- Modified wheat starch
- Oats (some experts say oats can be safe when certified gluten free but in general it is wise to avoid oats or any oat derivative.)
- Oat bran
- Rye
- Seitan
- Semolina
- Spelt
- Triticale
- Wheat
- Wheat bran
- Wheat germ

- Wheat starch

Other possible sources that should be questioned:

- HVP/HPP (Hydrolyzed plant or vegetable protein)
- Modified food starch
- Dextrin
- Maltodextrin
- Starch

Foods that contain gluten (unless specifically gluten free):

- Pasta
- Noodles except rice noodles and mung bean noodles
- Breads and pastries including cornbread and potato bread, naan, pita, etc.
- Crackers including pretzels and graham crackers
- Most cereals and granolas including corn flakes, rice krispies and rice puff (They contain malt which contains gluten.)
- Breading and coating mixes
- Dressing and stuffing
- Most sauces and gravies
- Flour tortillas and some corn tortillas
- Malt beverages including beers, largers and ales
- Granola bars and energy bars

Foods to be cautious of as they may contain gluten:

- Soy sauce – some contain wheat
- Bbq potato chips and some other potato chips
- Processed lunch meat
- Soup, especially cream soups such as cream of mushroom and cream of chicken
- Pickles (some of them have wheat derivatives)
- Bleu cheese (some are made using wheat and gluten)
- Hot dogs (some fillers contain wheat)
- Bouillon cubes (some contain wheat and gluten as thick

Items That May Contain Hidden Gluten:

- Imitation crab
- Seasoning packets
- Natural flavorings
- BBQ sauces
- Salad dressings
- Hard candies
- Ice cream
- Chipotles in adobo sauce
- Yogurt and sour cream (some use wheat or other glutens as thickeners)
- Miso
- Some fermented kimchi

- Fish sauce
- Oyster sauce
- Mole
- Beverages such as sports drinks or ice tea mixes
- Oats – oats need to certified GF and some people with celiac disease still have sensitivity to oats. Oats in processed foods like chili are not GF and should not be eaten on a GF diet.

Other items that could contain gluten:

- Some multigrain tortilla chips
- Marinades
- Brown rice syrup (It is sometimes made with barley.)
- Meat substitutes like veggie burgers, vegetarian sausage, imitation bacon and any other imitation seafood. They often contain a protein called seitan made from gluten.
- Starch or Dextrin in a meat product, it could contain gluten
- Pre-seasoned or marinated meats found in the butcher's area of the grocery store or in the meat case
- Cheesecake fillings, some contain wheat flour
- Eggs at some restaurants, which have added, pancake batter to make the eggs fluffier
- Flavored coffees and teas
- Some chocolates
- Imitation bacon bits
- Candies such as licorice

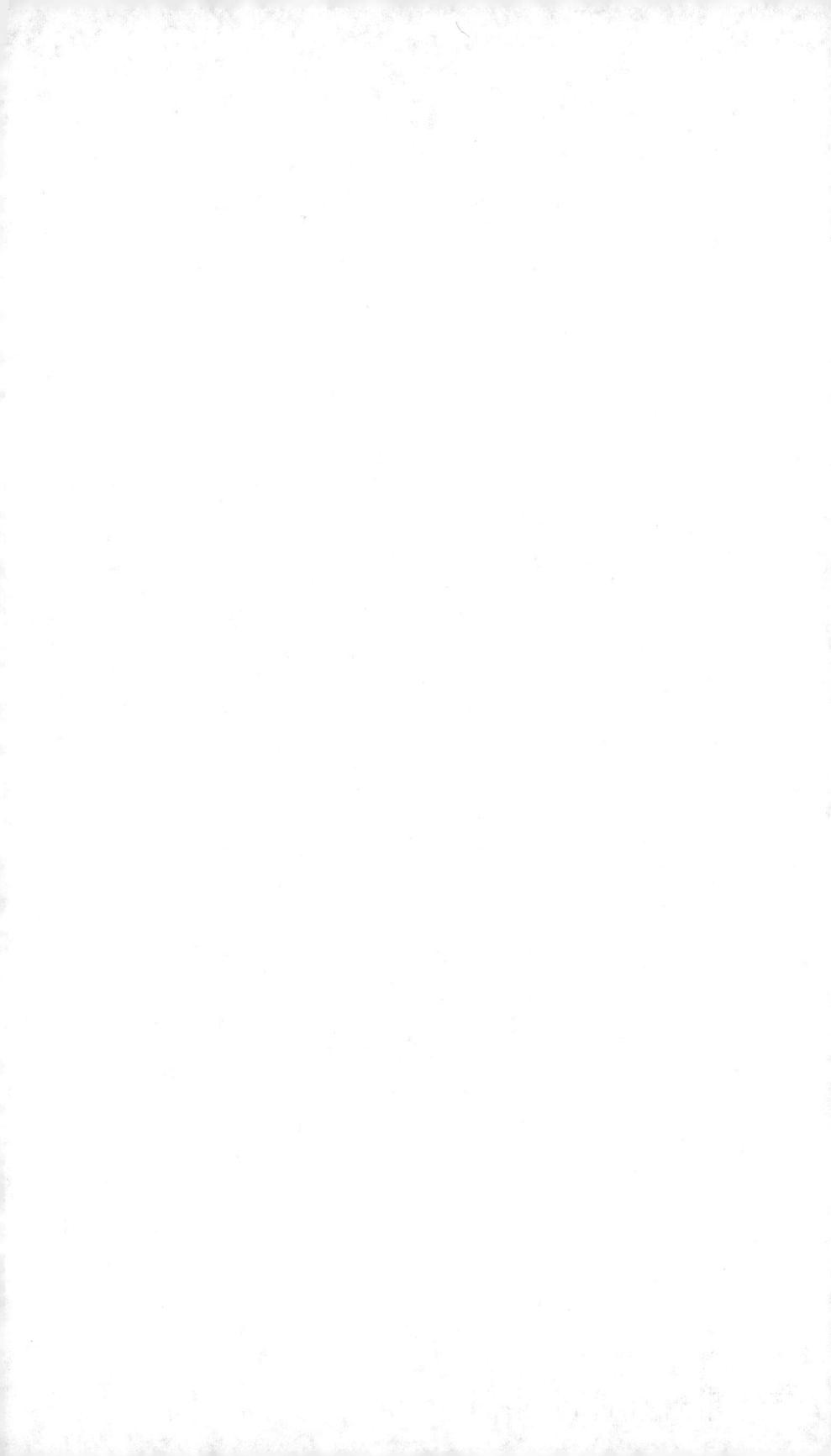